THE HEALTHY PROSTATE

A Doctor's Comprehensive Program for Preventing and Treating Common Problems

Arnold Fox, M.D.
and
Barry Fox, Ph.D.

John Wiley & Sons, Inc.
New York • Chichester • Brisbane • Toronto • Singapore

To our wives, Hannah and Nadine,
who make all things possible.

This text is printed on acid-free paper.

Library of Congress Cataloging-in-Publication Data

Fox, Arnold
    The healthy prostate : a doctor's comprehensive program for preventing and treating common problems / Arnold Fox and Barry Fox.
        p.   cm.
    Includes bibliographical references and index.
    ISBN 0-471-11982-2 (pbk. : alk. paper)
    1. Prostate—Diseases—Popular works.   I. Fox, Barry.   II. Title.
    [DNLM: 1. Prostatic Diseases—prevention & control—popular works.
    2. Prostatic Diseases—therapy—popular works.   WJ 752 F791h 1996]
    RC899.F69   1996
    616.6'5—dc20
    DNLM/DLC
    for Library of Congress   95-24189

10 9 8 7 6 5 4 3 2 1

Trademarks

Achromycin is a registered trademark of Lederle Laboratories
Amikin is a registered trademark of Bristol Laboratories
Augmentin is a registered trademark of Beecham Laboratories
Azactam is a registered trademark of E.R. Squibb & Sons, Inc.
Bactrim is a registered trademark of Roche Laboratories
Cardura is a registered trademark of Roerig
Cefizox is a registered trademark of Smith Kline & French Laboratories
Cefobid is a registered trademark of Roerig
Ceftin is a registered trademark of Allen & Hanburys
Ceptaz is a registered trademark of Glaxo Pharmaceuticals
Cipro is a registered trademark of Miles, Inc.
Claforan is a registered trademark of Hoechst-Roussel Pharmaceuticals, Inc.
Cleocin is a registered trademark of The Upjohn Company
Coumadin is a registered trademark of DuPont Pharma
Cytadren is a registered trademark of CIBA-GEIGY Corporation
Donnatal is a registered trademark of A.H. Robins Company
Duricef is a registered trademark of Mead Johnson Pharmaceuticals
Eulexin is a registered trademark of Schering Corporation
Garamycin is a registered trademark of Schering Corporation
Geocillin is a registered trademark of Roerig
Hytrin is a registered trademark of Abbott Laboratories
Lupron is a registered trademark of TAP Pharmaceuticals, Inc.
Macrobid is a registered trademark of Procter & Gamble Pharmaceuticals
Maxaquin is a registered trademark of G.D. Searle and Company
Mefoxin is a registered trademark of Merck Sharp & Dohme
Mezlin is a registered trademark of Miles, Inc.
Minipress is a registered trademark of Pfizer Laboratories
Motrin is a registered trademark of The Upjohn Company
Nalfon is a registered trademark of Dista Products Company, a division of Eli Lilly
Nebcin is a registered trademark of Eli Lilly and Company
Netromycin is a registered trademark of Schering Corporation
Nizoral is a registered trademark of Janssen Pharmaceutica, Inc.
Noroxin is a registered trademark of Merck Sharp & Dohme
Omnipen is a registered trademark of Wyeth-Ayerst Laboratories
Orudis is a registered trademark of Wyeth-Ayerst Laboratories
Pen-Vee is a registered trademark of Wyeth-Ayerst Laboratories
Pipracil is a registered trademark of Lederle Laboratories
Primaxin I.V. is a registered trademark of Merck Sharp & Dohme
Proscar is a registered trademark of Merck Sharp & Dohme
Prostat is a registered trademark of Horizon Crest
Rocephin is a registered trademark of Roche Laboratories
Septra is a registered trademark of Burroughs Wellcome Co.
Tylenol is a registered trademark of McNeil Consumer Products Company
Vibramycin is a registered trademark of Pfizer Laboratories
Zoladex is a registered trademark of Zeneca

Contents

Introduction

The prostate has become hot news. Prostate cancer has grabbed the headlines by striking celebrities such as Jerry Lewis, politicians such as Bob Dole, and heroes like General H. Norman Schwarzkopf. Meanwhile, a less exciting but often devilishly painful enlargement of the prostate called benign prostatic hypertrophy has been quietly sending hundreds of thousands of men to their doctors' offices, looking for relief.

In the coming chapters we'll examine the prostate itself—how the various prostate ailments are diagnosed, the medicines, surgeries, and other therapies used for prostate problems—and then look at my Healthy Prostate Program. Armed with an understanding of the prostate gland, prostate drugs and surgeries, plus alternative approaches, you will be equipped to discuss with your physician any problems that may arise.

Although I strongly believe that all serious problems require attention, and that minor problems must be prevented from becoming major, I do not believe that strong medicines or surgeries are the answer to all prostate problems. I've seen many a "cure" that has turned out to be worse than the disease itself. I've also known many people who have refused treatment but fared very well. I'm not advocating that you ignore your doctor, however. Physicians are great for helping you discover what may be going wrong inside your body, as well as for suggesting treatments. But only you should make the choice to pursue strong medical or any surgical treatment. *Remember: All medicines and surgeries harbor some danger, and should be approached with healthy caution. Even a small chance of side effects may be too great if you're the one who has to live with them.*

How to Use This Book

Chapters 1 and 2 look at the physiology of the prostate and the surrounding area, then discuss the three main types of problems that strike the prostate. Chapter 3 delves into the diagnosis of prostate ailments. I suggest that you read these chapters in order. Then you may want to skip over to specific chapters, depending on your particular prostate problem. Chapter 4 looks at the main medicines used for prostate problems, Chapter 5 at the surgeries, and Chapter 6 at other treatments such as radiation therapy and "watchful waiting." Although you should read the chapter on surgery, for example, if you are seriously contemplating or scheduled for surgery, I urge you to read the chapters on medicine and other treatments as well, for you may find that another approach is better suited to your needs. Finally, even if you are comfortable with mainstream medicine, glance through Chapter 7. There you'll find brief discussions of some of the many alternative approaches to treating prostate problems.

Should you be given a diagnosis of prostate cancer, be sure to read Chapter 8, which presents the good and bad news about the cancer, describes how it is staged and graded, then describes my five-step approach to deciding what to do when faced with cancer. This unique approach guides you through a careful self-analysis that is a vital part of the thinking process you should undertake before making one of the most serious decisions in your life. I also encourage you to read Chapter 10, which is filled with the case histories of men who have been through the various prostate cancer treatments. We doctors can give you facts and figures, but there is nothing like hearing it from the "horses' mouths," the men who have already made the decision and enjoyed or suffered the consequences.

Whatever your prostate ailment or treatment, should you suffer from the common side effects of incontinence, sexual difficulties, or pain, read Chapter 9. There, you'll find suggestions for dealing with these physically and psychologically difficult complications.

The last main section in the book consists of Chapters 11 and 12, which describe my Healthy Prostate Program. In Chapter 11 you'll find ways to keep your prostate and immune system in tip-top shape. Chapter 12 outlines my treatment suggestions for prostate enlargement, infection, and cancer. Chapter 13 concludes the book with a very brief look at the latest information available as we went to press.

Should you come across a word you do not understand, look in the glossary for an explanation. Should you wish to find a self-help organization or a place to get more information, you'll find a list of resources in the Appendix.

My Thanks

I am indebted to many people who have helped me gather information for this book, including my son, Eric Miller, M.D., of Phoenix; Kathleen Cairns, Psy. D., of Beverly Hills, California; Douglas Chinn, M.D., of the Alhambra Hospital Cryosurgical Center of Southern California; James E. Pero, M.D., F.A.C.S., of Los Robles, California; Haim Bicher, M.D., the head of the Valley Cancer Institute in Los Angeles, California; Randy W. Martin, O.M.D., Ph.D., LAc., of Encino; Michael Krane, M.D., Medical Director of RadNet Management, Inc., in Los Angeles; Dr. Leonard S. Marks, of Los Angeles; Arnold Malcolm, M.D., of the Saint Joseph Medical Center in Burbank, California; and Nancy LaSota, R.N., M.N., Director of the CancerCare Program at Los Robles Regional Medical Center in Thousand Oaks, California.

Most of all, my thanks to my son and coauthor, Barry, who devoted countless hours to turning my often unorganized thoughts into a full-fledged book.

Arnold Fox, M.D.

1

The Prostate— An Overview of the "Unknown" Gland

A forty-two-year-old writer noticed that he had to go to the bathroom more and more often at night, but only a little bit of urine dribbled out each time. Even when he did have a full bladder, the urine came out very slowly. As he put it, "I could hardly make bubbles in the bowl anymore."

A thirty-seven-year-old teacher felt a little uncomfortable while urinating one morning. By the end of the day, he was almost doubled over in pain, absolutely unable to urinate at all.

A fifty-six-year-old businessman was dismayed at the results of the cancer surgery performed on his prostate. "They should have just cut off my penis entirely. It's worth nothing since the surgery."

These men, young men in their thirties, forties, and fifties, had prostate problems. Like most men, they had only the vaguest idea of where the prostate gland was, and what it was supposed to do. And like most people, they had thought that only old men had to worry about their prostates. Unfortunately, they were wrong. Prostate problems can strike at any age. Indeed, new diagnostic procedures are suggesting that younger men *have* been suffering from certain prostate problems all along, but we never realized it until now.

The word "prostate" comes from the Greek, meaning the gland standing before the bladder. Imagine that there's a small bucket sitting inside your abdomen—that's your bladder. A tube called the urethra comes from the bottom of the bladder and carries urine down through the penis and out of the body. Sitting right under the bladder, wrapped

1

around the urethra, is a walnut-shaped gland called the prostate. The prostate's primary job is to add fluid to the sperm as it comes up from the testicles and to expel it during ejaculation.

Unfortunately, the prostate is wrapped around the urethra, putting it in the perfect position to choke off the flow of urine from the bladder. When the prostate squeezes down on the urethra, or enlarges to push up against the bladder, or both, a man may have urinary—and possibly sexual—difficulties. He may feel the urge to go RIGHT NOW! but have to wait an agonizingly long time for the flow to begin. He may constantly dribble urine, suffer from ill-defined pain, and/or have urinary infections. He may be tired all the time because he has to get up to go to the bathroom five or six times a night. And many of these men may find sex to be difficult or impossible.

All of these effects are the result of the malfunctioning of a little gland that's just supposed to help sperm search for an egg to fertilize!

COMPLEX PROBLEMS WITH COMPLEX SOLUTIONS

Some historians have argued that World War II was caused by prostate problems. When World War I ended in 1918, the Allied leaders gathered in France to negotiate a peace treaty with the vanquished. But the victorious heads of state were old, and many had severe prostate problems. They couldn't sit for very long—certainly not through the interminable speeches and negotiating sessions. The theory is that they hurried through the treaty-making and botched the job, thereby setting the stage for World War II.

Of course, the average man isn't holding the fate of nations in his hands, but he undoubtedly would prefer to be able to sit through an entire movie, sleep through the night, or go for a Sunday drive without having to map out all the rest stops.

Although most doctors have a fair understanding of prostate infections and BPH (benign prostatic hypertrophy), we haven't established firm guidelines for diagnosing and treating these two problems. There's no agreement as to which tests should be used, in what order, and for what reason. As an experiment, I once sent a man to several different urologists—doctors who specialize in treating the urinary tract in men and women, and the male genital tract. Although the patient described the exact same symptoms to each of the doctors, each gave a different diagnosis, different prescriptions, and called for different tests. The urologists were all competent physicians; the differing diagnoses simply show how complex prostate problems can be. And the situation grows even more complex when prostate surgeries are considered. Men must choose from among the very popular TURP (transurethral resection of the prostate), TUIP (transurethral incision of the prostate), TULIP (transurethral ultrasound-guided laser-induced prostatectomy), BALDI (balloon dilation), LP (laser prostatectomy), MIC-HYP (microwave hyperthermia), VLAP (visual laser ablation of the prostate), TUNA (transurethral needle ablation), and cryo (freezing) surgery. In addition, special "braces" called stents can be placed into the urethra to hold it open. Which surgery or procedure is best? A man must choose carefully, for the wrong surgery may leave him incontinent (unable to hold his urine) or impotent (unable to maintain an erection). Even the "right" surgery, perfectly performed, can have unfortunate results. And in some cases, no surgery is the best choice, because every surgery carries with it the risk of death.

To assist—and complicate—matters further, pharmaceutical companies offer many medicines for prostate infections and BPH. The different drugs work in different ways and on different aspects of prostate problems. However, they all have powerful side effects, which may include dizziness, lack of energy, weakness, sleepiness, nasal congestion, decreased sexual desire, and impotence.

Meanwhile, the alternative health community is offering various vitamins, minerals, pollens, amino acids, fatty acids, and other substances to solve prostate problems. Excellent double-blind, crossover studies done at hospitals and universities around the world have shown great results from certain alternative BPH thrapies, while others do nothing. Some physicians and other healers point to the power of the mind-body connection as a way of stimulating the body's defenses against prostatic infection and other problems.

As if prostate infections and BPH were not enough, prostate cancer is also on the rise: It's now the second most common cancer for men. Actors Bill Bixby and Telly Savalas, singer Frank Zappa, and Nobel laureate Linus Pauling are among the men recently felled by prostate cancer. General H. Norman Schwarzkopf, who led Allied troops through the 1991 Persian Gulf War, has had surgery for prostate cancer. Junk-bond king Michael Milken found out that he had prostate cancer the day he was released from prison. The tests, treatments, drugs, surgeries, and alternative therapies for this disease are numerous and diverse. Surgery can be helpful, but many men have been left totally incontinent or impotent as a side effect of prostate surgery. Yet, other prostate cancer patients, who have had absolutely

---

Early Ideas on the Causes of Prostate Problems

A 1903 book titled *The Nonsurgical Treatment of Prostatic Disease* presented the following reasons for prostate disease:

> *Men are by nature much more sensuously inclined than women: and when they cultivate libidinous impulses and associate with prostitutes, are liable to indulge their sexual propensities to such an extent as to develop passions that may lead to grave moral vices, like excessive intercourse or masturbation resulting in lesions of the prostate. . . . [D]iseases of the prostate gland cause such various forms of mental disorders as inactivity, depression, and numerous other neurotic aberrations.*

In those days, it was quite common to blame prostate problems on sexual overindulgence. In 1905, however, a book called *Enlargement of the Prostate: Its Diagnosis and Treatment* pointed out that, while sexual misbehavior may lead to prostate problems, it's also possible that prostate problems may prompt sexual misbehavior:

> *From the enlarged and tender prostate of the young masturbator, to the similar organ of the old man who married a young wife—it has been common to blame the sexual excitement as the efficient cause; but . . . it is probably quite as logical, if not more so, to blame the enlarged prostate with exciting unnatural desires.*

Today, of course, we know that neither of these learned arguments is correct.

---

no treatment at all, live long, healthy lives. As far as the ten-year survival rate is concerned, it doesn't seem to matter much which treatment one chooses—or whether one has any treatment at all. But should a man take the chance of forgoing treatment? And how does he make the right decision?

The problems, the proposed solutions, and the confusion will continue to grow as more and more men enter the "prostate years," and as more drugs, surgeries, procedures, and alternative therapies come into use. Men—and those who care about them—will be faced with many hard choices concerning a little gland of which, at best, they previously had only a vague awareness. Let's put the prostate in perspective by taking a brief look at the male reproductive system. Then we'll discuss the much publicized gland itself—what it is, what it does, and why it so frequently malfunctions.

A MAN'S ANATOMY AND PHYSIOLOGY

Figure 1.1 gives you an overview of the area we'll be talking about in this book. At the top of the figure is one of two kidneys that sit on either side of the body, a little bit below the lungs. Urine produced by the kidneys flows down through the two ureters into the bladder, then into the urethra as it travels through the penis and out of the body. Right below the bladder and above the penis is the prostate.

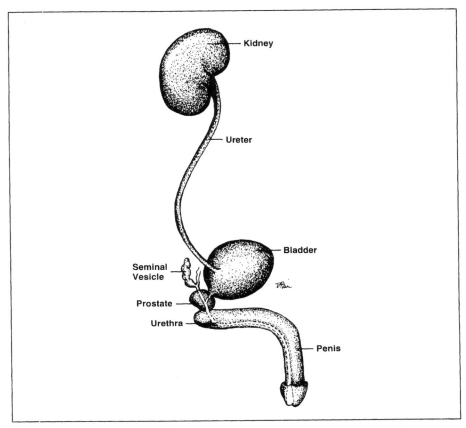

FIGURE 1.1 A side view of the male anatomy. *Drawing by Dawn Buie.*

Although the male reproductive system is quite straightforward compared to its female counterpart, it is made up of quite a few tubes, glands, and ducts squeezed into a relatively small space. Since there's no room to build the male ejaculate in a single location, the sperm must travel a circuitous route from station to station as the final ejaculate material is put together.

Inside each of the testicles, some 700 to 800 feet of tubes, called seminiferous tubules, are coiled around and about. These seminiferous tubules make up about 90 percent of the mass of the testicles. It takes approximately seventy-four days for spermatogenesis (the time required to make a sperm). Other parts of the testicles either provide nutrients for the developing sperm or secrete testosterone (the male hormone).

Sperm moves from the seminiferous tubules into a series of ducts that take it into the epididymis. The thin epididymis, like the seminiferous tubules, is a pair of long, coiled structures, one sitting astride each testicle. Sperm collects in the epididymis, maturing and waiting until needed (see Figure 1.2).

From the epididymis, sperm moves into the vas deferens—two heavily muscled, small tubes that coil up and around the bladder to the two seminal vesicles, which sit underneath the bladder, toward the rear. The seminal vesicles are essentially factories that produce and then store a nutrient-rich fluid that nourishes sperm as it travels out of the man's body when he ejaculates.

About the Testicles[1]

The word "testicles" comes from the Latin *testiculus,* which is a diminutive of the Latin word *testes,* meaning witness. The testicles were considered to be witnesses, or proof, of virility. Under Roman law, no man was allowed to testify as a witness or to vote unless he was able to demonstrate his manhood by proving that his testicles were present.

The word "orchis" has been used to identify the testicles since ancient days. The beautiful orchid is so named because its roots are shaped like testicles. At one time, the orchid root was used on patients with diseased testicles.

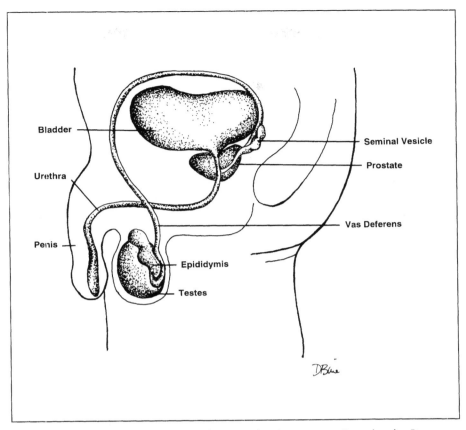

FIGURE 1.2 A side view of the male reproductive system. *Drawing by Dawn Buie.*

From the seminal vesicles, the road map of the male reproductive system takes us into the prostate, a walnut-shaped gland sitting directly beneath the bladder. The additional fluid generated by the prostate helps nourish the sperm as it travels through the woman's body in search of an egg to fertilize.

During a man's orgasm, muscles in the testes, epididymis, and vas deferens contract in concert, sending sperm into the urethra. Muscles in the seminal vesicles and prostate gland also contract, adding their fluids to the mix. When the urethra is filled with sperm and fluid, muscles at the base of the penis contract, causing ejaculation.

ABOUT THE PROSTATE

The prostate in a newborn male is about the size of a pea, gradually growing to about the size of a chestnut and weighing just under an ounce in an adult male. Normally, unless infection strikes, the prostate remains quiet until the average man is in his forties or fifties, when BPH sets in and it begins to grow again. We don't know why the prostate grows in an adult male, because the growth serves no discernible purpose. In fact, the new growth often makes men uncomfortable, and can become dangerous, or even deadly (see Figure 1.3).

Imagine a very small, walnut-shaped gland sitting beneath your bladder: That is the prostate. The urethra, in addition to transporting sperm, carries urine out of the bladder, down through the middle of the prostate and into the penis. The urethra running through the prostate is called the *prostatic urethra*. The external sphincter muscle sitting at the base of the prostate is the muscle a man uses to voluntarily control his urine.

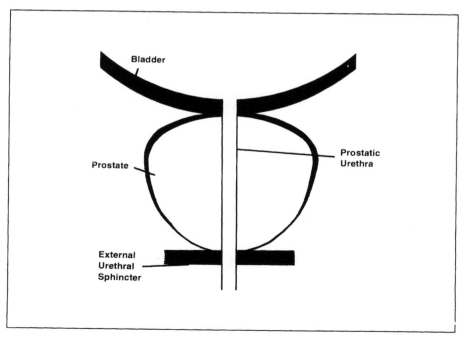

FIGURE 1.3 A stylized drawing of the prostate. *Illustration by R. C. F.*

The prostate itself consists of glands and ducts embedded in muscle fibers. The glands secrete fluid that passes through the ducts to join with the sperm in the urethra, forming the semen. In fact, sperm accounts for only about 5 percent of a man's semen. The rest is composed of seminal and prostate fluid. Muscle surrounding the prostate contracts during orgasm, helping to push the sperm/fluid mixture down the urethra.

That, in brief, is the prostate gland: simple and straightforward. A small gland produces a fluid that mixes with the sperm, and then it helps to push the semen/fluid along by contracting at the appropriate time. So how can it cause so much trouble to so many men? Chapter 2 provides a closer look at BPH, prostatitis, and prostate cancer.

2

What Can Go Wrong—and Why

There are three main types of prostate problems: infections, an overgrowth called BPH, and cancer. Infections of the prostate are common in men from their teens up. They can be mild or severe, long-lasting or quick to disappear. As men move into their late thirties and early forties, many begin to feel the unpleasant effects of an enlargement of the prostate called BPH (benign prostatic hypertrophy). Prostate infections and BPH can cause annoying, possibly dangerous, symptoms with far-reaching effects. The third type of prostate problem is cancer—a potentially deadly disease—yet most men who develop prostate cancer will not die of it. Indeed, many will die of other causes, never knowing that they had cancer. Let's begin with a look at infections of the prostate.

PROSTATITIS

It hit me little by little, so gradually that I hardly noticed it, the twenty-nine-year-old attorney explained. *Before it happened, I'd wake up every morning with a full bladder, and have one powerful pee. I'd slept the whole night through.*

About five years ago I had this girlfriend who had constant bladder and urinary tract infections. We only went together for a little while, but almost immediately I began getting up once a night to go to the bathroom, then twice, now three times every night. My stream seems to be all braided up, like some little girl's hair. It's weak, and it goes for a little while, it stops, then it goes again.

The problems come and go, but they never completely go away. I assume I got something from her, but who knows?

Like many men, this young attorney has prostatitis (inflammation of the prostate). Prostatitis is a common problem accounting for the complaints of as many as 25 percent of all men visiting their doctors with genitourinary problems.[1] Men are at increased risk for prostatitis if they have abnormalities in their urinary tracts, have had recent or recurrent bladder infections, engage in anal intercourse (active partner), or have recently had a medical instrument inserted into their penises.

Technically, "prostatitis" means an inflammation of the prostate gland, but doctors in the past have given the diagnosis of prostatitis to men complaining of a wide variety of problems in the area below the navel. Pelvic pain, lower back pain, perineal pain, and testicular discomfort have all been diagnosed as prostatitis. So have difficulties with urinating, gaining or holding erections, and ejaculating. In other words, prostatitis has been a catchall diagnosis for many diseases and discomforts that could not otherwise be diagnosed. Recently, however, prostatitis has been divided into four types: acute bacterial prostatitis, chronic bacterial prostatitis, nonbacterial prostatitis, and prostatodynia.

Acute Bacterial Prostatitis

The least common type of prostatitis, acute bacterial prostatitis is a sudden and/or serious inflammation of the prostate caused by bacteria. Often afflicting young men, it may be caused by *Escherichia coli,* *Klebsiella, Pseudomonas,* or other germs.

John is a forty-two-year-old marketing executive who enjoys excellent health. A former high school and college track star, he exercises often, watches his weight, and eats "lots of vegetables and fruits." Although deadlines and pressure to "score a big deal" make his job stressful, John makes it a point to "leave the problems at the office," to meditate thirty minutes every day, and to spend a full day every weekend with his family. "All in all," he says, "I've got a great life." However, one morning when he had gone to the office as usual, feeling fine:

> *By ten or so I was feeling sort of odd. I had a pain that wasn't really a pain about two inches beneath my belt and two inches in; I felt almost nauseous, but not really; I thought the heat was up because I was a little sweaty. My secretary said I looked a little ill, but I didn't think much of it.*

It hit me during lunch. It was like all my insides beneath the belt tightened up; I couldn't stand up straight. I was walking around like Igor the hunchback, dragging a leg. I felt hot, then cold. I was sick.

John's acute bacterial prostatitis hit hard and fast. In a general sense, acute bacterial prostatitis is like any other major bacterial infection in the body, but it happens to be localized in the prostate. (Had the infection settled in John's stomach instead of his prostate, he might have suffered bouts of vomiting and diarrhea.) As with other infections that have entered the blood, the bacteria may produce both fever and chills, as well as a general sense of malaise. In addition, because the infection is centered in the prostate, men may have pain anywhere "beneath the belt," all the way through to the back and down to the genitals. There may also be urinary difficulties such as urgency, frequency of urination, incomplete voiding of the bladder, even a complete inability to urinate. One patient described acute bacterial prostatitis as "like having BPH *and* the flu at the same time."

The process by which a man gets bacterial prostatitis is the same as with other infections: Bacteria entering the body are not destroyed by the immune system. Instead, they "settle down"—in this case, in the prostate. The infection may have arrived through the urethra, or perhaps it spread from an infection elsewhere in the body via the bloodstream. In order to make the diagnosis of acute bacterial prostatitis, the doctor will note the general symptoms (such as fever, chills, pain) and insert a finger into the patient's rectum to probe the prostate. The prostate may be enlarged, hard, irregularly shaped, or tender. If the doctor "massages" the prostate with a finger, the prostatic fluid can be pushed into the urethra and out the tip of the penis (or it can be flushed out of the urethra upon urination). Subsequent microscopic examination of the prostatic fluid may reveal the offending bacteria. *Note: Vigorous prostatic massage is* not *recommended, for it may cause the bacteria to spread.*

Acute bacterial prostatitis is usually treated with antibiotics and bed rest, plus intravenous fluids and other measures as necessary. Some of the medicines used include Bactrim (timethoprim/sulfamethoxazole), Septra, Cipro (ciprofloxacin), intravenous aminoglycoside, and ampicillin sodium. Most cases respond well to treatment. If unchecked, acute bacterial prostatitis can lead to abscesses in the prostate, problems with the seminal vesicles or epididymis, a blood-borne infection called septicemia, or chronic bacterial prostatitis.

Chronic Bacterial Prostatitis

It's the craziest thing, Doctor Fox, lamented fifty-two-year-old Arthur, a construction foreman. *For a couple weeks I'm running to the bathroom all the time, and then for a while I have no problems. For a couple weeks I have to wait a long time to start peeing, and then the problem disappears for a while. But it always comes back. It's been coming back for years now.*

Like the acute version, chronic bacterial prostatitis is an inflammation of the prostate caused by bacteria. But the chronic form generally produces few symptoms, and lasts much longer. Apparently, the bacteria settle into the prostate for a long stay, or return again and again. The immune system prevents the germs from spreading too far or doing too much damage, but it can't seem to get rid of them entirely.

Diagnosing chronic bacterial prostatitis can be difficult because the symptoms are generally less severe. The man may suffer from urgency, frequent urination, excessive nighttime urination, pain upon urination, or difficulty urinating. The symptoms may lessen or disappear for a while, only to blossom and return again.

The fact that the man has the same infection over and over again is an important diagnostic clue. When the doctor uses a finger to examine the prostate, it may feel perfectly normal, or it may feel inflamed. The doctor will likely massage the prostate in order to expel prostatic fluid through the urethra. The fluid will then be examined in the laboratory. If there are more than ten to fifteen white blood cells per high-power field, prostatitis is a likely cause.[2] (White blood cells are immune system "soldiers" that rally to fight infection. The presence of more white blood cells than normal suggests that the immune system has gone to battle.)

Chronic bacterial prostatitis is usually treated with antibiotics such as Cipro (ciprofloxacin), Maxaquin (hydrochloride), and tetracyclines. But while the drugs are good at knocking out acute bacterial infections, they're not as effective against chronic prostatitis because they don't penetrate well into the prostate. Interestingly, some experts recommend that men with chronic bacterial prostatitis regularly empty the ducts and glands of their prostates by ejaculating frequently (through either sexual intercourse or masturbation).

With improvements in ultrasound techniques in the past several years, doctors are beginning to find stones (calculi) in the prostates of many patients with chronic bacterial prostatitis. Some experts feel that these stones "shelter" or encourage infections. If this is true, one solution would be to remove the stones surgically.

Nonbacterial Prostatitis

The third form of prostatitis is nonbacterial: Bacteria do not seem to be involved, although the symptoms are similar to those of bacterial prostatitis. Laboratory examination of fluids massaged out of the prostate may show an increased number of white blood cells, suggestive of a problem of some sort, but bacteria can't always be found in the samples. Either bacteria are not the cause, or some bacteria that elude identification are responsible.

Although we don't know what causes nonbacterial prostatitis, we do know that it is often found in younger, sexually active men, often following a case of nonspecific urethritis (urethral irritation caused by nondetectable bacteria or by nonbacterial means). This suggests that whatever caused the problem was transmitted sexually.

We don't know exactly how to treat nonbacterial prostatitis because we don't know what causes it. Some patients seem to benefit from antibiotics, but trying any old medicine to see what works is not a good idea. Neither is long-term antibiotic therapy, for that can damage the body. As with chronic bacterial prostatitis, increased frequency of ejaculation seems to help some nonbacterial patients.

PROSTATODYNIA

A twenty-five-year-old actor came to my office complaining of pain in the midgroin area. The pain was worse when he had an erection.

"Doc," he said, "I'm young, and I really enjoy sex. But now I just can't do it." He had been seen by urologists in Beverly Hills and Los Angeles, but had not been helped by the medicines they had prescribed. My own examination plus a review of his records produced no significant findings, so I treated him with a Swedish pollen extract called Prostat. He soon felt fine, later calling me to report that he had "upheld" his reputation.

Although prostatodynia is usually grouped together with prostatitis, I separate it because most cases of prostatodynia probably do not involve the prostate. Prostatodynia refers to pain that appears to come from the prostate, or the area around the prostate. However, many patients with prostatodynia also have back pain or other back prob-

Problems in Close Proximity to the Prostate

A lot of interconnecting glands, tubes, and ducts are packed into a relatively small space in and around a man's genitals. Problems in one area can quickly affect, or spread to, another.

Urethritis—An inflammation of the urethra. Since part of the urethra (the prostatic urethra) runs through the prostate, the symptoms of urethritis may be confused with the symptoms of prostate problems. Urethritis may be caused by an adjacent infection, such as in the bladder or kidneys. Doctors may prescribe antibiotics and pain medications while trying to identify and treat the offending organism(s).

Epididymitis—An acute or chronic inflammation of the epididymis (the two long, coiled ducts, one sitting atop each testicle, that carry sperm from the testicles to the vas deferens). Epididymitis may be caused by prostate surgery, prostatitis, an infection in the urinary tract, and certain sexually transmitted diseases. Doctors treat the underlying cause of epididymitis (if apparent), and may prescribe pain medication, scrotal support, and bed rest, as appropriate.

Orchitis—An inflammation of one or both of the testes. The inflammation may be caused by an infection, or by other diseases such as mumps, tuberculosis, or certain sexually transmitted diseases. Symptoms often include tenderness, swelling, and pain. Doctors treat the symptoms of orchitis with pain medications, cold packs to reduce the swelling, and by recommending that the man wear a jockstrap to support his testicles. The doctor may also treat the underlying disease or problem (if apparent).

Urethritis, epididymitis, and orchitis can strike singularly or in combination, with or without affecting the prostate.

lems, and there may or may not be urinary and sexual difficulties. The pain of prostatodynia may be due to an inflammation of the muscles of the pelvic floor, spasms of the urethra, or sclerosis (hardening) of the neck of the bladder. It's also possible that the underlying problem may be one of several anal and rectal problems, bladder cancer, extensive

calcification of the prostate, interstitial cystitis, or even prostate cancer. I've often seen prostatodynia in marathon runners and bicyclers,
triathletes, weight lifters, and even truck drivers who regularly drive
long distances.

There is no single treatment or cure for prostatodynia. The key is
to find the real cause of the symptoms, and proceed accordingly.

BENIGN PROSTATIC HYPERTROPHY (BPH)

Ralph, a sixty-two-year-old furniture salesman, came to my office
complaining of "pain." At least, that's what he told my receptionist
and nurse: He was too embarrassed to admit that he had urinary
difficulties.

> *I can't talk about that kind of thing with a woman,* he explained
> when we were seated alone in my office. *But I can tell you,
> man to man, my hose just isn't working anymore. It goes on and
> off when it wants to, not when I tell it to.*

Ashamed to admit that there was anything wrong with his "male
equipment," Ralph had refused to see a doctor as his problem grew
worse over a twenty-year period. By the time I saw him, he was literally
in diapers, unable to control the constant drip of urine. Like millions
of other men, Ralph has benign prostatic hypertrophy, known as BPH
for short. BPH is an extraneous, *noncancerous* growth of the prostate.
("Benign" means noncancerous.)

We do not fully understand the reasons why male hormones cause
the typical man's prostate to begin swelling sometime in middle age,
although the enlargement can begin earlier. Autopsy studies of men
who have died prematurely for other reasons have shown that BPH can
affect men as young as twenty-five or thirty, and that 10 percent of the
men in this age group may have prostatic enlargement.[3] Some 50
percent of men aged sixty, and 90 percent of men eighty-five or older,
will have BPH. It's felt that almost every man will eventually develop
microscopic evidence of BPH, if he lives long enough.

Although BPH is widespread, it was usually ignored in the past
because there wasn't much that could be done about it. Now, with
new medicines and surgeries, treating BPH has become a booming
mini-industry for doctors, especially urologists. Each year, BPH accounts for some 1.7 million visits to doctor's offices, and surgeons are

busy operating on about 400,000 prostates yearly. Surgical care for the prostate alone costs the United States three to four billion dollars annually.

We doctors still don't know for sure how men get BPH. It may be that evolution failed to give us good mechanisms to keep the prostate under control as we age. According to that theory, once men have successfully donated their sperm in the reproductive process, both they and their prostates are superfluous.

What Happens When the Prostate Becomes Enlarged

Although we don't know why men develop BPH, we do know what happens when the prostate grows beyond its limits. Remember that the urethra passes right through the center of the prostate, carrying urine out of the bladder and down through the penis. As we said in Chapter 1, the part of the urethra that goes through the prostate is called the *prostatic urethra*. Prostatic tissue is wrapped completely around the prostatic urethra, but it has only a gentle grip on the vital tube. Below the prostate is the external urethral sphincter, the muscle that men voluntarily contract to hold back urine. As BPH begins to develop, overgrown prostatic tissue (shaded in Figure 2.1) begins growing around

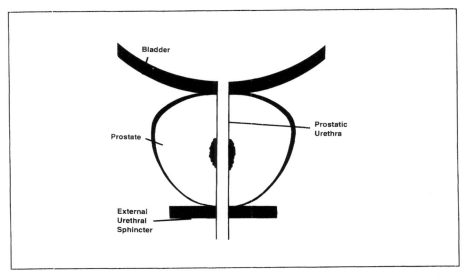

FIGURE 2.1 A prostate with minor BPH pressing against the urethra. *Illustration by R. C. F.*

the prostatic urethra. It begins as a small growth, barely squeezing against the urethra.

The BPH may remain relatively small or may continue growing, tightening its grip on the urethra and possibly interfering with the urinary flow (see Figure 2.2).

Should BPH continue, it can become like strong hands squeezing a throat, choking off the flow (as shown in Figure 2.3). With BPH throttling the urethra, a man may find it difficult to urinate, despite a great urge to do so. As a result, many men at this stage find themselves waiting and waiting for their stream to begin, wondering what's wrong. The flow may also be weak. As one patient put it, "I really had to go, but it took forever to start. And then it had no force."

Not all men actually notice a problem, especially if their symptoms have crept up slowly. They simply may not remember that their urinary streams used to begin immediately, remaining at full force until the end, or that they once could fill the bowl with bubbles.

If BPH continues, it may completely shut off the flow of urine through the prostatic urethra. At this point, urinating is a difficult task; urine is likely to pool in the bladder, increasing the risk of infection. "Back pressure" from the bladder to the kidneys may even result in

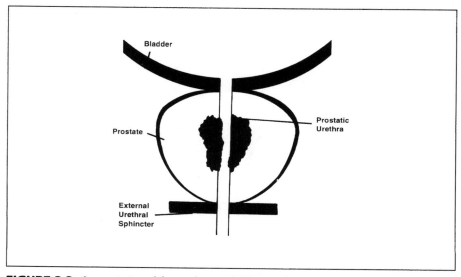

FIGURE 2.2 A prostate with moderate BPH pressing against the urethra. *Illustration by R. C. F.*

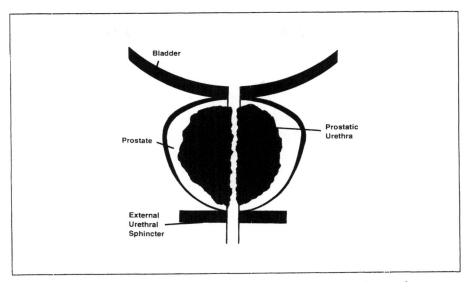

FIGURE 2.3 A prostate with significant BPH pressing against the urethra. *Illustration by R. C. F.*

kidney damage. In some cases, BPH clamps down on the prostatic urethra *and* pushes up against the bladder, wreaking havoc on the poor man's urinary system, as illustrated in Figure 2.4.

Symptoms of BPH

Let's take a look at some of the symptoms of BPH and their causes and effects.

Hesitancy in urinating or straining to start

Starting the stream of urine can be difficult if BPH is causing the prostate to squeeze down upon the prostatic urethra. The bladder muscles, which contract to push urine out of the bladder and into the urethra, have to exert extra pressure to force the urine through the partially or significantly narrowed urethra.

A weak urinary stream

Like other muscles in the body, the muscles surrounding the bladder grow when exercised. (In this case, the "exercise" consists of trying to push urine out of the bladder through a narrowed prostatic urethra.)

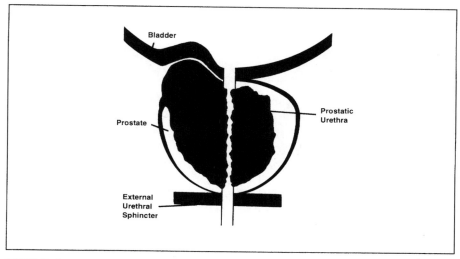

FIGURE 2.4 A prostate with significant BPH squeezing the urethra and pressing against the bladder. *Illustration by R. C. F.*

Unfortunately, unlike muscles in your arms or legs, bladder muscles become "disorganized" and inefficient if forced to grow too much. The muscles, which at first handled the extra work by growing a bit, eventually weaken. With weaker muscles pushing urine through the system, the urinary stream loses force.

Starting and stopping

As with a weak stream, a urinary flow that starts and stops is due to problems with the bladder muscles. Instead of being able to shoot the urine all the way through the urethra with one strong contraction, the bladder gives several weaker pushes as it struggles to expel its contents bit by bit.

Dribbling

With a healthy system, the urine stream starts almost immediately, it remains at full force until almost the end, and only a few drops remain in the pipes to be quickly squeezed out. When BPH strikes, however, small amounts of urine may remain in the bladder or urethra awaiting one final, weak push from the bladder muscles. Unfortunately, that last push may come *after* a man has pulled up his zipper, resulting in a wet spot on his underwear.

Frequent urination

A part of the bladder called the trigone sits on the floor of the bladder, right inside the bladder neck. Very sensitive to the presence of urine, the trigone signals the brain that it's time to urinate when it comes in contact with sufficient amounts of liquid. And as the bladder muscle builds up in response to BPH, the trigone becomes even more sensitive. As the sensitivity increases, the trigone develops a hair-trigger response, signaling the need to urinate when only relatively small amounts of urine are present.

Urgent urination

When there is a need to go RIGHT NOW!, there is no waiting until the movie is over, or until you get home. Like frequent urination, urgency is due to buildup and oversensitization of the bladder.

Nocturia

Nocturia means excessive nighttime urination, specifically having to awaken from sleep to urinate. Men often notice the extra nighttime trips to the bathroom before they notice any daytime changes. It's annoying to be awakened by the call of nature, so we're aware of even one extra trip to the bathroom at night. Furthermore, there's nothing to distract us from that urge when we're sleeping, as there is during the day when we're busy with work and play. Nocturia leads to daytime fatigue.

Incomplete urination

Weakened by the struggle to push urine into a constricted prostatic urethra, the bladder may not be able to empty itself completely. Some urine may always remain. This can lead to frequent urination as the never-empty bladder quickly refills. In severe cases, a man may have to urinate every thirty minutes or so. There may also be infections fed by stagnant urine, as well as involuntary leakage, blood in the urine, and other problems.

Incontinence

In highly advanced cases of BPH that lead to severe bladder damage, a man may have difficulty controlling his urine at all.

BPH itself does not trouble men. The overgrown cells could sit unnoticed in the prostate forever if they didn't press upon the prostatic urethra and the bladder. But if BPH continues unchecked, it *may* lead to bladder infections that spread to other parts of the body, to kidney damage, or other problems. But there are few absolute rules with BPH. Many men have no discomfort despite what seems to be significant BPH. Others are driven to distraction by relatively mild BPH.

BPH symptoms are classified as being either *dynamic* or *static*. Dynamic symptoms, involving the smooth muscles of the prostatic urethra and the bladder neck, can change rapidly as the muscles contract or relax. Static symptoms, caused by the overgrowth of prostate tissue, are slow to change.

Do You Have BPH?

There are no hard-and-fast guidelines to help us determine who has BPH, and to what degree. But the following exercise, based on the American Urological Association's Symptom Index, can help us arrive at a standardized approach to BPH. For each of the following seven questions, circle the number that best describes your situation. Add the numbers you circle to get your total score.

BPH Symptom Index

	Not at all	Less than 1 time in 5	Less than half the time	About half the time	More than half the time	Almost always
1. During the past month, how often have you felt like your bladder was not completely empty when you finished urinating?	0	1	2	3	4	5
2. During the past month, how often have you had to urinate again less than two hours after you last urinated?	0	1	2	3	4	5
3. During the past month, how often have you found that you stopped and started again several times during urination?	0	1	2	3	4	5
4. During the past month, how often has it been difficult for you to postpone urination?	0	1	2	3	4	5
5. During the past month, how often have you had a weak urinary stream?	0	1	2	3	4	5

	Not at all	Less than 1 time in 5	Less than half the time	About half the time	More than half the time	Almost always
6. During the past month, how often have you had to push or strain to get your urinary stream started?	0	1	2	3	4	5
7. During the past month, how many times have you typically arisen at night to urinate?	0	1	2	3	4	5

Add the numbers you've circled to get your Total Score _____ . If your score is 0–7, you probably have no, or only mild, BPH symptoms. If your score is 8–19, you probably have moderate BPH symptoms. If your score is 20 or more, you probably have severe BPH symptoms.

Treating BPH

There are many treatments for BPH. The approach called "watchful waiting" consists of keeping a careful eye on the situation, but holding off on strong medicines or surgeries until it's clear that they are really needed. Medical treatments include the use of drugs such as Proscar and Hytrin (see Chapter 4). Surgical treatments for BPH include transurethral resection of the prostate, transurethral incision of the prostate, transurethral laser-induced prostatectomy, hyperthermia, balloon dilatation, stents, and coils (see Chapter 5). Alternative treatments include the use of various herbs and other preparations (see Chapter 7).

Knowing the alternatives, you might ask, "Which treatment is best?" There is no right answer. What's best for you depends on the severity of your BPH, the symptoms, your past medical history, and other factors. The best approach is to investigate the various treatments, and to discuss the appropriate course(s) of action with your physician.

CANCER OF THE PROSTATE

Some two hundred thousand American men will be diagnosed with prostate cancer this year; comedian Jerry Lewis is but one of the many men who have already been given the sad news. Thirty-eight thousand American men will die of cancer of the prostate this year. Yet, as scary as prostatic cancer sounds, many victims will die never knowing that they had it, for one can live quite well with the disease. In fact, of those men now harboring prostate cancer, the majority will die of other causes.

Prostate cancer is the second most frequently diagnosed cancer in men (after skin cancer), and it is the second most frequent cause of cancer deaths in American males[4] (behind lung cancer). However, the incidence of prostate cancer is actually much higher than some statistics of diagnosis indicate. Autopsy studies of men who have died of various other causes suggest that 30 percent of all men over the age of fifty have undetected cancer of the prostate. It may not be bothering these men, but it's there. By age ninety, the majority of men who died for other reasons will have autopsy findings of cancer of the prostate.

Cancer of the prostate is popularly considered to be an "old man's problem," something that happens to men age fifty and up. But is fifty old? I used to think so. I used to believe that thirty was old. Now that I'm in my sixties, I no longer think of fifty as old. Thanks to advances in nutrition, sanitation, and medicine, a fifty-year-old man can expect to live many more years today.

The symptoms of prostate cancer can be a big problem, but not because they're so painful. The difficulty is that there are often no symptoms at all, or only very minor ones, during the early stages of the disease. With no pain, discomfort, or other warning signals, a man often has no idea that anything is wrong. The first symptoms a man notices are usually very similar to those of BPH, including:

- Nocturia—getting up at night to urinate, often frequently
- Frequency—urinating frequently, but often only small amounts
- Hesitation—having to wait longer for the urine flow to begin
- Intermittency—a start-and-stop flow of urine

It should be pointed out that having these symptoms *does not prove* that a man has prostate cancer. But if they are present, it's a good idea to see a doctor for a thorough workup of the prostate, in the hopes of ruling out cancer. This is especially important when you remember that 30 percent of all men over the age of fifty have the disease.

Although prostate cancer begins in the prostate gland, it does not always remain in place. That's the biggest concern, because one can live reasonably well with a diseased prostate, or even no prostate at all. The greatest danger comes when the cancer outgrows the gland and invades other organs. It may eat its way into the bladder or hitch a ride in the bloodstream. Likely, it will take up residence in the nearby pelvis, the lumbar spine (lower back), the femur (thigh bone), the thoracic spine (mid- and upper back), or the ribs. With a more advanced spread, the cancer may paralyze the lower extremities by pressing against the spinal cord, but luckily, this does not happen often. There's even the possibility—rare but nonetheless real—that the cancer may spread to the liver, lungs, or brain. Perhaps most unfortunately, by the time that almost half of all prostate cancers are detected, they have already spread beyond the prostate.[5] They can be treated, yes, but because they have spread, they are considered incurable.

How Do You Get Prostate Cancer?

Cancer should not be the serious problem that it is, for the human immune system is designed to destroy cancerous cells. In fact, it's theorized that we all have small episodes of cancer many times in our lives, but that our immune systems quickly destroy the cancers before they cause any trouble. If we do develop a cancerous condition that spreads, it is because the cancer has overwhelmed, eluded, or outsmarted our immune systems. Generally speaking, the stronger a person's immune system, the lower the risk of cancer. Unfortunately, many of us go through life with weakened immune systems due to many causes, including:

- Hereditary factors
- Stress
- Exposure to various chemicals
- Poor nutrition

Sooner or later a cancer may overwhelm our natural defenses and take hold. Although we don't know exactly why men get prostate cancer, we do know that there are two steps involved in the transformation of an ordinary cell into a cancerous one: *initiation* and *activation*.

Initiation

DNA (deoxyribonucleic acid) serves as the "instruction manual" for every single cell in the body, telling the cells exactly what to be and what to do. A part of those instructions directs the cells to cooperate with each other to keep the body healthy. For example, a cell is supposed to grow only to a certain size, to take limited amounts of nutrients out of the common larder, and to produce so many daughter cells. Trouble arises when the instructions are somehow altered and a normal cell becomes *initiated* to cancer. Initiation is brought about by carcinogens (agents that cause cancer) such as ultraviolet light, radiation, cigarette smoke, and certain chemicals. Certain substances in food are also carcinogens, including fat, sodium, nitrate (used in curing meats), and the blackened portion of charbroiled foods.

Although initiated, the cells with the altered DNA are still harmless, and may remain quiet for days or decades. The initiated cells are willing and waiting to be bad, but they won't act until prompted.

Activation

Also known as "promoters," activators are instigators that stir initiated cells into cancerous action. Once they're activated, cancer cells multiply without restraint, gobbling up more than their share of nutrients from the bloodstream, crowding, invading, and strangling other parts of the body.

Initiators and Activators

There are many initiators and activators that, working together, can turn quiet cells into deadly cancer. They include:

Excess dietary fat

One of the most dangerous of agents, fat is both an initiator and an activator. Most scientists now agree that the standard, high-fat American diet contributes to or causes many cancers, especially the so-called cancers of affluence. The cancers of affluence are so named because people living in wealthy countries and eating high-fat diets get them much more than do those living in poor countries and eating low-fat diets. But it's not just rich people who eat high-fat diets; even less affluent people in richer countries tend to consume large amounts of fat.

The cancers of affluence include cancers of the prostate and pancreas in men, cancers of the breast, ovaries, and uterus in women, and cancers of the colon and rectum in both men and women. Various studies suggest that excess dietary fat is responsible for some 40 percent of the cancer deaths in men and 60 percent in women—quite a price to pay for the privilege of eating a high-fat diet.

Tobacco

Tobacco has long been known to be cancer-causing. Some one-third of cancers in the United States and Europe are related to tobacco use, especially to cigarettes and chewing tobacco.

Chemicals

Ample evidence has implicated various chemicals, such as benzapyrene and arsenicals, as well as others found in smog. In fact, a large swath of New Jersey has been called "cancer alley" because of the high cancer rates among those living in the area, where so much toxic waste was dumped. There have even been cases of adenocarcinoma of the intestine caused by a single asbestos fiber. A single fiber! That's how toxic some substances can be.

Sunlight

The wonderful sunlight that warms and tans us can also scramble the DNA inside many of our skin cells, putting us at risk for cancer. Four hundred thousand of us will develop skin cancer this year. Melanoma—the deadliest form of skin cancer—is on the rise.

Radiation

Radiation was first recognized as a cause of cancer not too long after the X ray came into use as a diagnostic tool in 1895. Doctors exposed to the X rays from those primitive machines began developing cancers of the skin on their hands and in other areas. There were also cancers among the young factory women who painted radium on the faces of watches so that the dial could be read at night. The workers kept pressing the brushes between their lips to keep them sharp, not knowing that they were taking in minute amounts of radiation all day long.

Is Prostate Cancer Genetic?

Researchers at the Johns Hopkins Oncology Center in Baltimore have recently reported that a "genetic flaw that inhibits a cell's ability to detoxify environmental carcinogens may be closely linked to the development of prostate cancer."[6] The researchers hypothesize that a certain enzyme in prostate cells may be accidently "turned off," leaving the cells more vulnerable to cancer-causing agents. If this idea is confirmed by further study, a test for the enzyme may be developed as a way of predicting which men will develop the cancer.

Are We Winning the War against Prostate Cancer?

According to the National Cancer Institute, the five-year relative survival rates for prostate cancer increased from 66.7 percent in 1974 to 77.6 percent during 1983–1989.

The "Best" and "Worst" States for Prostate Cancer

Geography *seems* to play a role in cancer mortality, as these cancer mortality statistics from 1987 to 1991 suggest. The reasons for the differences between the states are many and complex, including the age and race of the population and the availability and use of health-care services. Here are the four states with the highest rates of death due to prostate cancer, followed by the four states with the lowest rates. (Washington, D.C., is considered a state for purposes of this ranking.)

State	Rate (per 100,000)	Rank
District of Columbia	44.3	1
South Carolina	31.9	2
North Dakota	31.0	3
North Carolina	31.0	4
New Mexico	22.7	48
West Virginia	22.3	49
Alaska	22.0	50
Hawaii	16.0	51

Source: SEER Cancer Statistics Review, 1973–1991; U.S. Department of Health and Human Services; Public Health Service; National Institutes of Health.

Although the survival rates have improved in recent years, many researchers question whether this gain is significant. Yes, the absolute numbers are better, but they may be a result of our ability to diagnose cancer at earlier stages than we could ten years ago. We don't really know if the increase in survival time is due to surgery and other treatments, or simply due to early detection.

Treating Prostate Cancer

There are several approaches to treating prostate cancer, including surgery, radiation, freezing, and alternative ideas. We'll look at medical treatments in Chapter 4, at surgical approaches in Chapter 5, at radiation, heat, and hormonal treatment in Chapter 6, and at alternative ideas in Chapter 7.

3

How Prostate Problems Are Diagnosed

Back in the 1950s, there were few tools to assist in diagnosing prostate problems. Placing a finger in a man's rectum allowed physicians to palpate his prostate, but specific blood tests and imaging were many years in the future. We often could not diagnose prostate cancer until it had spread painfully through a man's body, and by then it was too late.

We've come a long way since then, and now we have a wide variety of diagnostic tests and procedures that can help us diagnose prostate problems. This chapter covers the tests that should be done and the order in which I recommend they be performed. If you suspect you have a prostate problem, this information will help you by preparing you for what may happen when you see the doctor.

THE "MUST DO" TESTS TO DIAGNOSE PROSTATE PROBLEMS

Regardless of your age, race, or symptoms, every initial examination should include a detailed discussion of your personal, family, and medical history, and a digital rectal examination (in which the doctor inserts a finger into the rectum in order to feel the prostate).

Must Do Test #1: The "Talking Test"

During the many years that I taught physical diagnosis to medical students and residents, I emphasized that every examination must begin with a conversation, for talking to a patient provides 90 percent of the information needed to make a diagnosis. That's right: Simple conversation and intelligent questioning are excellent diagnostic tools.

29

Whether you are seeing your doctor for a routine examination or are there because of specific problems, the visit should begin with a friendly grilling—as your physician asks you many questions about yourself, as well as your medical and family history. Asking about your past medical history, learning what illness and surgeries you've already had and what medicines you are taking, can alert your doctor to potential problem areas.

Knowing what you do for a living and how you spend your free time can also be helpful. For example, in my experience, men who work with chemicals have a higher rate of prostate and bladder problems than do other men. In addition, learning about your family is important, for men whose fathers have had prostate cancer may be at greater risk for the disease than those whose fathers have not.

It is vital that every doctor question male patients about possible problems with the prostate, for many men are reluctant to volunteer that information. Indeed, an October 1991 Gallup Poll revealed that over 60 percent of men who already had prostate problems had not discussed their difficulties with their doctors.[1] There are many reasons for this: (1) Young boys are taught that "real men" never complain, (2) many men are reluctant to admit to any problems in the genital area, and (3) quite a few men think that such problems strike only the elderly, and they believe that admitting to such problems means that they're over the hill.

Jim's case history illustrates the importance of thorough questioning: He was a fifty-seven-year-old truck driver, a muscular "man's man" who complained of back and stomach pain. "But the back pain is from lifting," he said, "and the stomach pain is probably ulcers. Don't you think it's ulcers?"

He might have had ulcers, but I went through my full questionnaire with him. Although he had checked "no" or "never" to all the questions regarding sexual or urinary problems, I asked him the same questions, in a slightly different way. Again, he denied any problems in those areas. "It's too much lifting and ulcers, doc. That's what it is."

As we continued talking, I asked him what he does on a typical day, how many boxes he lifts, what he eats, and so on. The answers surprised me. For one thing, he stated that since he had been assigned a new route three years ago, he only lifts a few very light boxes every day. It seemed a little odd that his back would hurt now, when he'd been lifting less than he had for years. Further, he told me that his bland diet had been the same for many years, and that his new route was the easiest, least-stressful run he had ever had. Unstressed men who eat bland foods can certainly get ulcers, but his answers weren't fitting the usual pattern.

Suspecting a prostate problem, I asked him if he usually filled the toilet bowl with bubbles when he urinated. Although surprised by the seemingly silly question, he answered "no." We kidded around about how, as boys, we used to fill the entire bowl with bubbles when we urinated, except for a small area around where the streams hit the water. We laughed as we remembered how we'd move the "no bubble" area around the bowl, and how we'd swish the stream back and forth across urinals. Relaxed, he dropped his guard and admitted, "I haven't been able to do that in years. Now I've got to wait forever for it to start, and it just kind of dribbles out."

It seemed clear that Jim had a prostate problem. As it turned out, he had a massive infection of the prostate, which was responsible for his back pain. He later confessed that he didn't have any stomach problems; he just couldn't bring himself to admit that there might be something wrong with his "equipment." So he told the doctors there was something wrong with his stomach, hoping they'd stumble upon the real disease.

That's why a good doctor will ask many questions, and then will ask the same questions again in a different way, in case the patient didn't understand or didn't want to reply to the probes as originally stated.

Questions and more questions

Your doctor must ask you if you've had any urinary or sexual problems, or any pain or other symptoms anywhere in your pelvic area, "belly," lower back, or sides. Try to be honest. But even if you say no, the doctor should continue asking specific questions, such as:

- How many times do you urinate during the day, on average? At night?
- Do you ever have to rush to get to the toilet on time?
- Do you ever leak urine before you get to the toilet? When you sneeze or cough?
- Does your urinary stream start right away, or do you have to wait? Do you ever have to strain to start the stream? To keep it going?
- On a scale of one to ten, with ten being very strong and one being a slow dribble, how would you rate the force of your urinary stream? Has the force changed recently? Over the past year? Couple of years? Many years?

- Do you start and stop when you urinate? If so, how many times, on average?
- Does your urinary stream turn into a dribble when you approach the end of a urination?
- Do you ever continue to urinate after you thought you were finished? Have you ever had urine drip into your underwear or pants after you've finished urinating and dressed? Do you wear any sort of diaper, pad, tissue paper, or other device because you leak urine?
- Do you ever have any pain when urinating? Any burning? Any strange or unusual sensation?
- Have you ever had any treatment for urinary problems? If so, what were the problems and the treatments? Have you ever had any kind of urinary problem that bothered you, but for which you did not seek help?
- Has anyone ever told you that you should see a doctor for your urinary problems? Has a friend with urinary problems similar to yours ever seen a doctor for those problems?
- Do your urinary problems annoy you? Do they interfere with your daily activities, or enjoyment of life? Would you be upset if your urinary problems never got better?
- Do you have sexual difficulties?
- Do you have any difficulties getting an erection? Keeping your erection?
- Do you have any pain or discomfort at any time during sex? Any pain in the belly, sides, or back at any time during sex?
- Does semen come out of your penis when you ejaculate? Do you seem to have more or less semen per ejaculation than you did before?
- Have you ever had any treatment for sexual problems? If so, what were the problems and the treatments? Have you ever had any kind of sexual problem that bothered you, but for which you did not seek help?
- Has anyone ever told you that you should see a doctor for your sexual problems? Has a friend with sexual difficulties similar to yours ever seen a doctor for those problems?
- Do your sexual problems annoy you? Do they interfere with your daily activities or enjoyment of life? Would you be upset if your sexual problems never got better?

A "yes," "maybe," "sometimes," "sort of," or any other positive answer to any of these questions should elicit more questions as the doctor helps you describe your signs and symptoms in the greatest possible detail. If you feel embarrassed talking about your sexual and urinary habits, just treat your conversation with your physician as you would any other test—unpleasant, perhaps, but helpful to both you and your doctor.

A word of caution

If your doctor asks you to fill out a questionnaire before seeing you, make sure that the right areas are covered on the form, and make sure that your answers are reviewed. (There are doctors who ignore the questionnaires they have their patients fill out.) Don't assume that just because you fill out a form, the doctor either reviews it or understands the significance of your answers. Insist on reviewing the questionnaire with your physician. Don't be afraid to say, "I want to go over my answers with you." If your physician is annoyed, or refuses, get a new one. Your health is more important than any doctor's time or temperament.

Must Do Test #2:
The Digital Rectal Examination ("Finger Test")

Despite great advances in medical technology, the time-honored digital rectal examination (DRE) is still an important diagnostic tool. The DRE is a "hands-on," careful palpation of the prostate. Inserted through the patient's rectum, the doctor's gloved index finger feels both the right and left lobes of the walnut-shaped prostate. This simple procedure tells the physician about the size and texture of the prostate, whether it is smooth or rough, soft or hard, symmetrical or irregularly shaped. The doctor can also make sure the prostate is somewhat moveable, as it should be, and that it is not bumpy, lumpy, or covered with a mass.

With a DRE, the doctor can tell if the prostate seems to be enlarged. (Bear in mind that prostates come in different sizes. Your prostate may be larger or smaller than average, so finding that your prostate is "larger than average" is not necessarily the same as finding that it is enlarged.) For comparison, it's best if the same doctor has examined your prostate in the past.

The doctor can also tell if your prostate seems to be bogey (squishy). A bogey prostate may indicate infection and inflammation.

Any sort of a bump or lump must be evaluated further. A definite, discrete, firm nodule, or a stone-hard gland (or part of a gland) generally indicates a significant risk of cancer. It's generally accepted that about 50 percent of hard, bumpy nodules or stone-hard glands may contain cancer. Also, there are other abnormalities a doctor may find—such as a local area of benign (noncancerous) enlargement, stones in the prostate, or even tuberculosis of the prostate.

Your reaction to the doctor's probing finger may also be a diagnostic tool, as it was in Mark's case:

> *"The doctor explained the finger thing, then did it. He slid it in a little and said, 'Does that hurt?'"*

> *"I said, 'no.'"*

> *"He slid it in some more and said, 'Does that hurt?'"*

> *"I said, 'no.'"*

> *"Then he pushed his finger against my prostate and said, 'Does that hurt?'"*

> *"When I finally came down from the ceiling, I said, 'Yeah, that hurt.'"*

Mark's prostate was very swollen and very painful. The slightest touch sent "lightning bolts of pain all the way out my penis," as he put it. Mark's doctor was able to measure his progress not only by the way his prostate felt in later examinations, but by how much pain Mark felt when the doctor felt his gland.

How a DRE is done

The DRE is quick and simple. I ask the man to lower his pants and shorts, then lean forward and over the examination table. I have plastic gloves on both my hands. After spreading his cheeks with my left hand, I gently insert my right index finger, which is lubricated, into the man's rectum, my palm facing the patient's left side. Then I turn 45° to the left, so my finger is on top of the prostate. My finger sweeps over the entire gland, left to right, comes down the median ridge (the groove separating the right and left lobes), and finally, gently over each lobe. The entire DRE takes less than a minute. It is awkward for men, but usually not painful.

How often should a DRE be performed?

With the development of new tests, many doctors are saying that the DRE is no longer necessary, or at least not very important. Critics point out that the DRE alone is not always sufficient to rule out cancer, for several reasons, including:

- The DRE is subjective. What one doctor thinks is abnormal, another may overlook.
- Not all prostates feel alike. They vary in how smooth, firm, round, and mobile they are from man to man, making the diagnosis difficult.
- Not all cancers feel cancerous; some cancerous growths may feel quite "normal" for a long time. Small growths may not be detected at all.
- Not all of the prostate can be felt with a DRE. If the cancer is in a nonaccessible area, it cannot be felt.

Perhaps I'm a bit old-fashioned, but I believe that the hands-on, digital rectal examination should be performed yearly for men over the age of forty. If any abnormality is found on the digital rectal, or if the patient has unexplained symptoms such as back pain, a prostatic ultrasound and a PSA should also be done. Someday, we may have a small, inexpensive machine that will "look into" the patient's body with 100 percent accuracy. Until then, I believe we doctors should keep doing DREs. There is no substitute for a supportive, unhurried physician who touches, and cares about, patients. Touching and caring are powerful medicines.

Although neither the Talking Test nor the DRE can provide all the answers, together they give the doctor and patient a lot of information, and help guide the rest of the examination. These two tests must be a part of every initial examination.

BLOOD TESTS TO DIAGNOSE PROSTATE PROBLEMS

There are six blood tests commonly used in the diagnosis of prostate problems: the PSA, the (RT)-PCR, the serum acid phosphatase, the alkaline phosphatase, the BUN, and the creatinine. We'll look at each of these tests in this section.

Before taking any of these or other tests, tell your doctor which (if any) medications, supplements, or other pills or potions you are taking. Also, ask if you should do anything special in preparation for the test(s).

Blood Test #1: PSA

Someday, people may look back upon the early 1980s as the beginning of a new era in medical diagnosis, for that is when the PSA test was made available by pharmaceutical companies. The PSA, a simple blood test, measures the levels of Prostate Specific Antigen in the blood. Prostate specific antigen (PSA) is a substance produced by the prostate. The higher the level, the greater the *possibility* of prostate cancer. The PSA rises when a man has cancer because:

- Cancer can cause the prostate to grow larger, and, generally speaking, larger prostates produce more PSA than do smaller prostates.
- Cancerous prostate cells make more PSA per gram than do non-cancerous prostate cells.

It should, therefore, be a simple matter of measuring the PSA levels in the blood to diagnose cancer. Unfortunately, it's not quite that easy, because:

- If you have a small prostate with a low PSA level, adding cancer to the equation may only bring your PSA up to "normal."
- If you have a large prostate with a relatively high PSA level, the test may suggest that you have cancer when you are, in fact, healthy.
- Prostate infections can make the PSA go up.
- BPH can make the PSA go up.
- The prostate drug Proscar (finesteride) can make the PSA go down,[2] possibly masking the presence of cancer.
- A primitive—but still very malignant—cancer may not be making much PSA yet.

That's why the PSA can tell us only if there is reason to suspect cancer, not if the cancer absolutely does or does not exist.

Until recently, most physicians agreed that PSA levels below 4.0 ng/ml are "safe"; levels between 4.0 and 10.0 are suspicious, and levels above 10.0 are considered very suspicious. Now we're beginning to use more specific, age-adjusted PSA levels. Unfortunately, we haven't yet forged a universal agreement as to what the age-adjusted levels should be. Here's one authority's proposal:[3]

Age Range	Healthy Serum PSA
40–49	2.5 or less
50–59	3.5 or less
60–69	4.5 or less
70–79	6.5 or less

The age-adjusted PSA numbers will undoubtedly change before there is general agreement as to a final configuration.

Take Your Tests in Order

If you are undergoing tests for prostate problems, pay close attention to the order in which those tests are performed. According to
a study reported in the *Journal of Urology*, PSA levels can rise when
the doctor uses a needle to take a biopsy (sample) of prostate
tissue.[4] Thus, the PSA test should be done *before* a needle biopsy.

Although the same study reported that DRE, prostatic massage, and ultrasonography have only "minimal effects" on serum
PSA levels in most patients, even a minimal change in PSA should
be avoided when possible. To be safe, I recommend that the PSA
test be performed first whenever practical.[5]

Refining the PSA

Researchers have come up with two methods for making the PSA a
more useful diagnostic test:

PSA Density. This is an attempt to eliminate the confusion caused by
the fact that prostates are of varying sizes. If the PSA is slightly elevated, the doctor may order a transrectal ultrasound, which, among other
things, helps to determine the volume (size) of the prostate. Dividing
the PSA by the prostate volume gives the PSA density, which is basically a look at how much PSA is produced "per ounce of prostate."

PSA Velocity. If your PSA is somewhat suspicious, the doctor may
have you return periodically for a repeat test. If the level rises over
time, a cancer may be growing and pumping out more PSA.

PSA density and PSA velocity can both help refine the diagnosis
and begin to point to the proper direction for further treatment.

Will PSA replace DRE?

Although the PSA is very valuable, a careful history and physical examination, plus the digital examination, should continue to be among
our medical tools. There have been countless times when the tip of a
gloved right index finger has led to the diagnosis of prostate cancer. It's
not high-tech, but it has saved many lives. In several studies comparing
the efficacy of the DRE and the PSA in detecting cancer, each has
proved to have its own limitations, and neither can detect or rule out

cancer in 100 percent of the cases. A combination of DRE and PSA remains most effective.

Blood Test #2: (RT)-PCR

As good as the PSA is at suggesting the presence of prostate cancer, it doesn't tell us whether the cancer is contained or has spread beyond the prostate—a critical issue that can drastically change the course of treatment. Cancer that's truly confined to the prostate can be entirely eliminated by surgically plucking the prostate out of the body. Once the cancer has spread, however, removing the prostate is of little or no value.

A new test, called the Reverse Transcriptase Polymerase Chain Reaction, or (RT)-PCR, helps determine if the cancer has escaped from the prostate. Whereas the PSA checks the blood for the presence of a substance made by prostate cells, the new test looks to see if the cancerous cells themselves are floating around in the blood.

The basic idea is simple. If the cancer is confined to the prostate, the odds are low that it will have shed some of its cells into the general circulation. But if the cancer has burst out of the prostate and pushed into the surrounding tissue, it's more likely to have shed cells into the bloodstream. According to Ralph Buttyan, Ph.D., Director of the Molecular Urology Laboratory at Columbia-Presbyterian Medical Center in New York, the test "has the ability to detect one cell in a million or more, so we don't need a lot of cancer cells in the circulation to find them."[6]

Blood Test #3: Serum Acid Phosphatase

The serum acid phosphatase (ACP), an older test that has been in use for a long time, also helps determine whether or not prostate cancer has spread beyond the prostatic capsule.

ACP is a simple blood test, producing values (results) ranging from roughly 0.5 to 1.9 units/l (depending on the methods and laboratory used). High ACP levels generally suggest that a tumor has spread beyond the prostate. The ACP may also rise with prostatic infarction, Gaucher's disease, and other conditions, so an elevated ACP by itself does not necessarily prove that the person has cancer. Recent prostate massage, rectal examination, or catheterization may affect ACP results. Since ACP levels should drop following treatment, the test is also used to see if the cancer has truly been eliminated.

Blood Test #4: Alkaline Phosphatase

Alkaline phosphatase is an enzyme involved with the bones, liver, and other parts of the body. The alkaline phosphatase test (ALP) may be used to help determine whether or not prostate cancer has spread to the bones. Depending on the laboratory, ALP levels range between 90 and 239 units/l in men. (Values for women are different.)

Although an elevated ALP suggests the possibility that cancer has spread, because there are other diseases that can cause a similar reading, a high ALP alone does not mean you have cancer. The ALP is used in conjunction with other tests when the doctor suspects that you have prostate cancer that has spread beyond the gland itself.

Many drugs that interfere with liver function can interfere with the ALP test, including barbiturates. Broken bones can also affect the outcome of the test.

Blood Test #5: BUN

The blood urea nitrogen (BUN) test is really for the kidneys, not the prostate. But because severe prostate problems can cause a "backup" of urine into the kidneys, it's a good idea to evaluate the kidneys when prostate problems are suspected. As a matter of fact, the BUN is a part of most routine blood panels.

The BUN measures urea nitrogen found in the blood. Most of the urea nitrogen should be filtered out of the blood by the kidneys, and passed out of the body in the urine. Elevated BUNs may be due to an impairment of kidney function, which in turn can be caused by obstruction of the ureter. Since an enlarged or diseased prostate may be responsible for the obstruction, your doctor should check the BUN as part of the routine examination for prostate problems. (Indeed, it should be done as part of a routine physical examination.)

Depending on the laboratory, normal BUNs range between 8 and 25 mg/dl (milligrams per deciliter). Low BUNs may be seen with advanced liver disease. With high BUNs, the doctor should consider acute or chronic kidney failure, as well as look for the cause.

Blood Test #6: Creatinine

Creatinine is a by-product of the normal breakdown of muscle. Like urea nitrogen, creatinine should be filtered out of the blood in the kidneys and passed out of the body in the urine. An elevated creatinine level suggests that there is something wrong with the kidneys.

Depending on the laboratory, the normal creatinine range should be between 0.8 and 1.5 mg/dl.

URINARY TESTS TO DIAGNOSE PROSTATE PROBLEMS

How often you urinate, and what happens when you do, can help the doctor assess the health of your prostate and other parts of the urinary system. Urinary tests are often used in the diagnosis of BPH.

In this section, we'll be discussing the Urinary Diary, the Frequency-Volume Chart, Urinalysis, and Uroflowmetry. These are not the only urinary tests your doctor may recommend, but they will give you an idea of the types of urinary tests that are used to diagnose prostate problems.

Urinary Test #1: The Urinary Diary

The Urinary Diary is not a test as much as it is a way of helping you to figure out exactly how much you urinate, when, and how "well" or "poorly" you do so each time. Some doctors and clinics have elaborate forms for you to fill out, but the Urinary Diary can be a simple listing such as this:

Wednesday, October 25, 1995

8:00 A.M.—Urinated; felt strong urge to go, weak stream, dribbled a lot at end.

9:00 A.M.—Urinated; weak stream, started and stopped twice, felt like there was more still inside.

9:15 A.M.—Urinated; just a little dribbled out.

11:00 A.M.—Urinated; a moderate amount of urine, mild burning.

The Urinary Diary helps the doctor to get a good picture of the patient's urinary habits.

Urinary Test #2: Frequency-Volume Chart

The Frequency-Volume Chart is an elaborated version of the Urinary Diary. Instead of simply keeping track of when you urinate, you also keep the urine itself, so it can be measured.

During the test, which usually lasts twenty-four hours, the patient is asked to note when he urinates, and to urinate into a container. This allows the doctor to measure how much is passed with each urination, and how much is passed during the entire twenty-four hours. There are many possible results, such as:

- A normal amount passed with each urination, and a normal total.
- A normal amount passed with each urination, but a high total passed per day. In this case your bladder may be fine, but you may have diabetes or another disorder prompting you to pass more fluid than normal.
- A large number of urinations, each producing a relatively small amount of urine. This suggests urgency, often seen with BPH.

Urinary Test #3: Urinalysis

The urinalysis is a standard part of the routine physical examination. Typically, the nurse hands you a little bottle or cup and asks you to step into the bathroom to fill it up. This is a simple, painless, relatively inexpensive test that can provide a wealth of information.

Urinary Testing Jargon

Here's the meaning of some of those words your doctors may throw around:

Average flow rate—The average amount of urine flowing out per unit of time.

Maximum flow rate—The greatest amount of urine flowing out. In other words, how much is flowing when your stream is at its strongest.

Voided volume—How much urine you produce.

Flow time—How long the stream keeps flowing.

Time to maximum flow—How long it takes for your stream to reach its maximum flow rate.

A urinalysis test does not give a diagnosis. Rather, it points to problem areas. (For example, excess sugar in the urine suggests diabetes.) As far as the urinary system is concerned, the urinalysis may show problems such as:

- Red blood cells, suggesting there is bleeding in the urinary tract. More than 0–2 red blood cells per high power field is a warning sign of anything from a mild bladder infection to cancer.
- White blood cells, suggesting an infection. White blood cells are part of the body's immune system, dying in huge numbers to fight off bacteria and other dangers. More than 1–3 white blood cells suggest an infection somewhere in the urinary tract.
- Protein, suggesting problems with the kidneys.
- Bacteria, parasites, or yeast cells, suggesting that the urinary tract has been invaded by "germs."

Clean catch

The best urine cultures use "midstream" or "clean catch" urine. To get midstream urine, the patient begins urinating into the toilet. After passing a few ounces, without stopping, he slips a collecting jar in place and urinates into it, making sure to save the last portion of his urine for the toilet.

Culture and sensitivity

If there is suspicion of an infection of the urinary tract, the doctor will place a small portion of your urine into a small dish that contains some nutrients. If bacteria are present, they will grow and can be identified. Meanwhile, many little discs, each dabbed with a bit of a specific antibiotic, may be placed on the bacteria to see which medicine is most effective against this particular infection. The test is called the "culture and sensitivity." "Culture" refers to growing the bacteria, "sensitivity" to seeing which antibiotics work the best.

Urinary Test #4: Uroflowmetry

Uroflowmetry measures the flow of urine in order to evaluate the lower urinary tract and to see if the bladder outlet is obstructed. Essentially, you urinate into a funnel attached to one of several types of devices. The device measures the average and maximum flow rates, the voided volume, the flow time, and so forth. The equipment used may be very complex, or relatively simple.

Depending on the type of equipment used, you may be asked to push a button, count to five, then urinate into a large funnel. When you finish urinating, you count to five and push the button again. The results of the test are plotted on a graph. The resulting "curve" helps the doctor come to a diagnosis.

Various medications can affect the results of the test. So can embarrassment (if you are not comfortable urinating in the presence of a doctor or nurse, or with having to urinate into a strange-looking machine). There must also be enough urine in your bladder to make the test valid. A full bladder is required, but you should not be made to wait until you absolutely *have* to go. Neither should you be distracted by being given instructions during the test.

INVASIVE TESTS TO DIAGNOSE
PROSTATE PROBLEMS

An invasive test is any test in which something is put into the patient's body. (Technically speaking, blood tests would also be considered invasive.) Because all invasive tests present some degree of risk, discuss the pros and cons of these tests with your doctor. Ask exactly why the test is to be performed, what might be discovered, and whether or not a less risky test can be used instead.

In this section, we'll take a look at prostatic massage, cystoscopy and urethroscopy, retrograde cystography and urethroscopy, voiding cystourethrography, and prostatic biopsy. These are not the only invasive tests your doctor may call for, but the explanations that follow will give you an idea of the types of tests used, how they're done, and their advantages and drawbacks.

Caution: The invasive and visualization tests discussed in this section and the next involve the use of instruments pushed into your body, X rays, anesthetics, and dyes. There is always *a risk when things are pushed into your body, when X rays are taken, and when anesthetics are used. Moreover, any test involving the injection or infusion of dye into your body is potentially dangerous. Many people suffer allergic reactions to dye. Insist that your doctor inform you of the possible problems before agreeing to any test. Make sure that you and your doctor discuss your allergies and any previous reactions you may have had to medications, dyes, anesthetics, or other substances.*

Invasive Test #1: Prostatic Massage

This is the simplest of the invasive tests. As with the DRE, the doctor inserts a gloved finger into the patient's rectum and "massages" the prostate. The goal is to push fluid out of the prostate, through the urethra, and out of the body. Some doctors will quickly catch the prostatic fluid on a slide as it drips out of the penis. Others will ask the patient to use his hand to hold his penis shut, then collect the fluid at once. The fluid is sent to the laboratory, where the technicians see if they can culture (grow) any bacteria.

A variation of this test, used by some in suspected cases of prostatitis, is to have the patient urinate into container #1, then into container #2. After a prostatic massage, the patient is asked to urinate into container #3. The amounts of bacteria in the containers are compared in an attempt to see if the prostate is harboring an infection, or if the infection is in other parts of the urinary tract. (The man urinates into the first container to clear away any urethral debris or germs. The urine in the second container would tell the doctor what organisms came from the bladder and/or prostate. The urine in the third container would have the greatest likelihood of containing organisms that came from the prostate only.)

Invasive Test #2: Cystoscopy and Urethroscopy

Cystoscopy is a very scary-sounding test that allows the doctor to actually see into a man's urethra and bladder. Luckily, it doesn't cause the degree of discomfort that most men fear. A cystoscope is essentially a long, thin tube, like a telescope, which is inserted, with an anesthetic, through the hole at the tip of the penis and into the urethra (see Figure 3.1). Depending on exactly what your doctor intends to do, which instruments are being used, your physical condition, and your concerns, the anesthetic may be a jelly placed into the urethra to dull the pain, a sedative, or regional or general anesthesia. There are lenses in the scope to enhance the doctor's view. The "front" end of the cystoscope, the part put into the penis, has a little light. The "back" end, the part the doctor holds, has a place for the doctor to look through, a tube through which to infuse fluid, and other ports through which to place different instruments. The older cystoscopes are rigid, the newer ones flexible.

The cystoscope is pushed into the urethra and up into the bladder. Any urine in the bladder can run out through the scope. This is

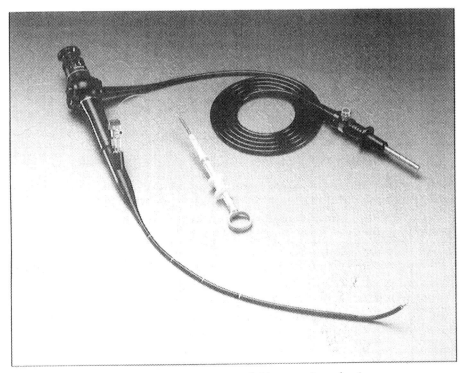

FIGURE 3.1 Cystoscope. *Photo courtesy of Olympus America Inc.*

very useful when the doctor wants to see how much urine remains in the bladder *after* you have finished urinating. (Ideally, the bladder should empty completely. We call what remains the "residual volume.")

Once any urine has been drained from the bladder, the doctor can infuse a sterile fluid through the scope into the bladder. This pushes the walls of the bladder back away from the "front" end of the scope, allowing the doctor to get a good look at the inside of the bladder. Cystoscopy allows the doctor to do many things, including:

- Measure residual volume, if any.
- Visually inspect the bladder and urethra.
- Gauge the degree to which the prostatic urethra is being "squeezed" by the prostate.
- Search for sources of bleeding, if any.

The cystoscope can also be used as a channel through which surgical instruments can be inserted into the patient's urinary tract. Minor surgical procedures, such as biopsies or dilatation of a constricted urethra, can be performed.

Urethroscopy is very similar to cystoscopy, but the examination is limited to the urethra. The same types of instruments are used.

Invasive Test #3:
Retrograde Cystography and Urethroscopy

Retrograde cystography uses a contrast medium (a dye) and X rays to make images of the bladder. "Retrograde" means backward. It is uncertain why the test is called a backward picture of the urethra, but possibly it is because the dye is injected up into the penis, opposite the normal flow of fluid.

For retrograde cystography, the patient is placed on an examining table and preliminary X rays are taken. A catheter is then threaded up the penis and into the bladder. A contrast medium is run through the catheter into the bladder, and the catheter is clamped off to hold the dye in place. With the bladder full of dye, X rays are taken from various angles. The catheter is unclamped, and the dye allowed to drain out. More X rays are taken with the bladder drained. In some cases, air may be injected back up the catheter, and X rays taken of the air-filled bladder. This is called the double-contrast technique, or double-contrast studies.

Retrograde cystography can help the doctor find tumors, stones, gravel, or blood clots in the bladder, diverticula (sacs or outpouchings in the bladder), and other problems.

Retrograde urethroscopy is very similar to retrograde cystography, using a contrast medium as well as X rays to make images of the urethra, rather than the bladder. The test may help the doctor find any problems in the urethra, including strictures, false passages, calculi (stones), and congenital abnormalities.

Invasive Test #4:
Voiding Cystourethrography

The purpose of this test is to look for abnormalities in the bladder and urethra, and possibly to detect hypertrophy of the prostate. The procedure is similar to a retrograde cystography, but now the patient is also asked to urinate so the doctor can get "pictures" of the voiding process in action.

With the patient lying on an examining table, a catheter is threaded into the penis and up to the bladder. A contrast medium (dye) is instilled through the catheter, filling the bladder, and the catheter is clamped off to prevent leakage. X rays are taken with the patient in various positions. Then the catheter is removed, and the patient urinates while more X rays are taken.

Invasive Test #5: Biopsy

Sometimes the doctor needs to examine an actual piece of your body to make a diagnosis, especially if cancer is suspected. Fortunately, very small pieces of tissue can be snipped out of the prostate with relatively little difficulty, pain, or danger.

The doctor may get the sample using one of three different routes:

- Perineal—A local anesthetic is given, and a small incision is made in the perineum (the area between the testicles and the anus). Using a finger to hold the prostate still, the doctor puts the biopsy needle through the incision to the prostate, and cuts off one or more small pieces of tissue.
- Transrectal—The doctor threads a needle through the rectum, pushes it through the thin lining between the rectum and the prostate, and removes some prostate tissue.
- Transurethral—The transurethral approach is generally used when the patient is undergoing cystoscopy or a similar procedure, and an instrument is already in place in the urethra. The needle is threaded through the instrument, then through the urethral tissue and into the prostate, and samples are taken.

If cancer is suspected, and depending upon the approach and the instruments being used, ultrasound is utilized to guide the doctor in putting the needle directly into the suspected nodule. The chances of getting a piece of the cancer tissue with the needle approach varies, with the skill of the physician and the extent of cancer being important factors.

A new procedure using a needle to draw some cells and fluid from the prostate (rather than a clump of tissue) has become popular lately. An experienced cytopathologist can then make the diagnosis by studying the fluid.

"VISUALIZATION" TESTS TO DIAGNOSE PROSTATE PROBLEMS

Visualization tests—especially the MRI—allow us to "see" into the body with an unprecedented degree of clarity. Although most people have not heard of the IVP, they may be familiar with the procedures used for ultrasound, kidney and bone scans, and MRI.

Visualization Test #1: IVP

The IVP (intravenous pyelography), also known as excretory urography, is an older test that was taught back in the 1950s, but it is not being used nearly as much now. The IVP allows the doctor to take a "picture" of the patient's kidneys, bladder, ureters (tubes connecting the kidneys and bladder), and other areas of the urinary tract.

For the test, a contrast medium (dye) is injected into one of the patient's veins. X rays or tomography allow the doctor to see where the dye goes, providing an idea of how well the kidneys, ureters, and bladder function. The patient's abdomen is pushed upon to move the dye through his urinary system.

The IVP can provide a lot of information about the kidneys, bladder, and ureters, but is not as useful for visualizing the prostate and urethra. The patient is exposed to a lot of radiation and is injected with a dye that can provoke mild to severe allergic reactions.

I do not recommend this test unless it is absolutely necessary and there are no alternative tests available. Many people suffer allergic reactions to dye, and even develop anaphylactic shock. Cardiac resuscitation has been required on patients who had bad reactions to the dye. Make sure your doctor knows about any allergies you might have, as well as previous reactions to medications, dyes, anesthesias, or other substances.

Visualization Test #2: Ultrasound

We've been using ultrasound techniques to image (see) various parts of the body for some time: in obstetrics (fetal ultrasound), for the heart (echocardiography), for the kidneys (renal ultrasonography), as well as for the gallbladder, ovaries, and uterus, among other applications. In women, the transvaginal ultrasound probe has helped us diagnose ovarian and uterine cancers, for example. Unfortunately, we couldn't get good pictures of the prostate until the mid-1980s. Now, thanks to new high-resolution scanners, we can get an "up-close look" at the prostate with transrectal ultrasound (TRUS)—a remarkably useful addition to our diagnostic capabilities.

Transrectal ultrasound delineates the normal and abnormal anatomy of the prostate, which makes it easier and quicker to diagnose cancer. Transrectal ultrasound not only measures the size of the tumor, it also gives us information regarding its possible spread.

Other Visualization Tests: Bone Scan and MRI[7]

Bone scans are used to help stage, not diagnose, cancer. That is, the tests are used to help determine whether the cancer has spread in men who have already been diagnosed. They may also be used for patients who have focal (localized) pain, and for other clinical reasons. Bone scans help determine whether or not the cancer has spread, because the bones are likely destinations for wandering prostate cancer (especially bones in the pelvis, hips, back, and upper legs).

The patient being scanned is given an IV (intravenous) injection of a radioactive material. After waiting for two to three hours, he lies down on a table while a special camera takes "pictures" of selected parts of his body. The picture-taking procedure takes half an hour to forty-five minutes.

The radiologist will later view the films, looking for "hot spots" that suggest cancer ("suggest" cancer, because the bone scan is sensitive but not specific). The test will detect "hot spots," but it can't tell you what caused them. (It may be cancer, but it may also be arthritis or an injury.) Doctors will use correlative X rays or other tests, as well as their clinical judgment, to expand upon the diagnosis.

Like the bone scan, the abdominal MRI (magnetic resonance imaging) is used only on men who have already been diagnosed as having prostate cancer. The test is used to help in local or regional staging of the cancer, to see how far it has spread before surgery or other treatment. It is not used to diagnose or screen prostate cancer.

For the test, the man lies on a pallet, a moving "tabletop" that slides in and out of the scanning chamber. An endorectal coil will likely be inserted into the man's rectum for part of the test, although there are new "phase array coils" that don't have to be placed in the rectum. The entire test takes thirty-five to forty minutes. Generally, during the scanning, the patient can listen to music, watch television, or chat with a friend or family member sitting nearby; he can even request sedation if frightened by the feeling of being enclosed. If a coil is to be inserted during the scan, the man will need a bowel prep (essentially an enema, which can be done at home).

The radiologist viewing the results of the MRI will look for alterations of anatomy, disruptions, nodules, enlarged lymph nodes, or other abnormalities. Because the patient is not exposed to radiation, and does not need to be injected with dye, the MRI is considered a very safe test. Unfortunately, it is also very expensive.[8]

THERE ARE NO SET PATHS TO DIAGNOSIS

You'd think that it would be simple to diagnose prostate diseases. Given the "Talking Test," the DRE, blood tests, invasive tests, and imaging tests, it should be an easy matter to pinpoint the cause of any problem. Unfortunately, no single test gives the doctor all the information necessary to make a definitive diagnosis. More than one test must be used, but there is no agreement as to which tests should be administered, and in what order.

As I mentioned in Chapter 1, I once experimented by sending a man to several different urologists. My "agent" described the same symptoms to each of the doctors, each of whom had a different approach to diagnosing prostate problems. All are good urologists. The differences in their approaches to diagnosis have to do with their personal preferences, what procedures and tests happened to be popular at the institutions in which they trained, what tests they've read about, and so on. Making a diagnosis is an art, not a science.

I cannot recommend which tests and procedures you should have. That's up to you and your doctor to decide, since every person's condition is unique. However, I tell my patients to take a slow but steady approach to diagnosis. Don't jump right to the exotic, expensive, and possibly dangerous tests—be a bit deliberate, and work your way up.

I always spend a lot of time on the "Talking Test" with my patients, as I have said previously. And I feel that a DRE is mandatory, whether I suspect the patient has prostatitis, BPH, or cancer.

If the patient's description of his problems is vague, I may request that he keep a Urinary Diary to help clarify the exact nature, timing, and extent of his symptoms. If I suspect BPH, I generally begin with a PSA and a "clean catch" urine culture to rule out cancer and prostatitis. If I suspect prostatitis, I usually begin with a "clean catch" urinalysis, and may massage the prostate to see if anything can be cultured from the prostatic fluid. If there is any reason to suspect cancer at that point, I may suggest a PSA and an ultrasound of the prostate. If these tests support the suspicion of cancer, I generally call for a biopsy.

These are only guidelines that I present to my patients at the early stages of investigation. You and your doctor may have other, equally valid approaches. Always bear in mind, however, that *you're* in charge. The doctor is only your adviser.

Now that we've discussed prostate problems in general, and their diagnosis, it's time to examine treatments.

4

Medicines for the Prostate

There are only a few main categories of prostate problems (BPH, prostatitis and prostatodynia, and cancer), but the diseases are quite different from each other, necessitating a wide variety of medicines. When I was a student and resident in internal medicine back in the 1950s, surgery was king of the prostate therapies. Today, we have many options, and the medical treatments are competing with the surgical for supremacy.

In this chapter we'll look at the medicines for BPH and prostatitis. Medicines and treatments for cancer are presented in Chapters 5 and 6.

MEDICINES FOR BENIGN PROSTATIC HYPERTROPHY (BPH)

There is no cure for BPH, that unwanted growth of the prostate that afflicts so many millions of men, with symptoms ranging from the very mild to the potentially deadly (in a very, very few cases). BPH is not a germ that can be knocked out. Neither is it caused by a lack of something that can be replaced by medication.

Although there is no "silver bullet" for BPH, no medicine that can quickly shrink the prostate or prevent it from impinging upon the prostatic urethra and bladder, medications are improving, and we may have a simple cure for BPH in the future. We do currently have two methods of partially relieving BPH symptoms with medicine: alpha blockade and androgen suppression. Let's look first at the alpha-blocking medications.

Alpha Blockade

Alpha blockade attempts to deal with the symptoms of BPH by encouraging certain parts of the prostate to relax, thereby lessening the pressure on the prostatic urethra, improving the urine flow, and reducing other symptoms.

Several alpha blockers have been used, are currently in use, and are being tested for future use, including Hytrin, Minipress, Cardura, and YM617. Hytrin is currently the more widely used alpha blocker.

Hytrin (chemical name: terazosin hydrochloride)

Description: Hytrin tablets contain the equivalent of 1 mg, 2 mg, 5 mg, or 10 mg of terazosin, plus several inactive ingredients. Depending upon the tablet, the inactive ingredients include cornstarch, lactose, talc, and dyes, among other substances.

Background: Terazosin was the first long-acting alpha blocker approved by the FDA for treating hypertension (high blood pressure).

How it works: In animal studies, terazosin reduces blood pressure by lowering the total peripheral vascular resistance. Simply put, this means getting the arteries to relax and open a little wider. Blood pressure equals the interaction between force (how much blood your heart attempts to push through with each beat) and resistance (how easily the blood flows through the pipes). If you reduce the resistance, the blood pressure drops.

Rationale: Why is a medicine for high blood pressure used to treat BPH? Some of the symptoms of BPH are caused by contraction (tightening) of the smooth muscle of the prostate. The smooth muscle contracts when certain substances interact with what are called the alpha receptors in the prostate. Alpha blockers such as Hytrin interfere with the alpha receptors, helping to keep the prostatic smooth muscle relaxed. It is hoped that the newly relaxed prostate tissue will move away from the urethra, relieving and reducing the pressure.

Hytrin is a "selective" alpha blocker, which means that rather than working on all the alpha receptors, it zeroes in on specific ones (the $alpha_1$ adrenoceptors). Selective alpha blockers tend to have fewer side effects than nonselective $alpha_1$ blockers because their action is more narrowly aimed.

Intended use: The medicine is intended to be used for those with high blood pressure, as well as for treating men who have *symptomatic* BPH. In other words, there must be enlargement *and* symptoms before the medicine is indicated. You should not be taking Hytrin just because your prostate is enlarged.

How well does it work? It works fairly well if the prostate symptoms are due to contraction of the smooth muscle, and not to enlargement of the prostate alone.

Who should not *take Hytrin?* This medication can be quite dangerous, and should be used cautiously. It should not be used by anyone who has low blood pressure, syncopal (fainting) spells, or dizziness.

Side effects: Side effects may include blurred vision, fainting spells, dizziness, light-headedness, palpitations, nasal congestion, nausea, peripheral edema, somnolence, weakness, drowsiness, and tiredness.

Effects on laboratory tests: Hytrin can upset the results of the standard blood test, significantly decreasing the hematocrit, hemoglobin, white blood cells, total protein, and albumin. Make sure that your doctor knows you are taking Hytrin and interprets your blood results accordingly.

Special warning: Beware of the "first-dose" effect. With the first few doses, Hytrin and other alpha blockers can cause large drops in blood pressure, which can result in syncope (fainting). This can also happen if you miss a few doses and then start taking the medication again. If you faint while standing, you may hurt yourself when you fall. If you're driving a vehicle or operating machinery when you faint, the results can be disastrous.

Avoid driving or doing any potentially dangerous tasks for at least twelve hours after taking your first several doses, after your dosage is increased, or after beginning to take the medicine again if therapy has been interrupted. Avoid any situation where dizziness or fainting could be hazardous. (Even holding an infant can be dangerous, if you should faint.) Should you feel dizzy, faint, light-headed, or otherwise "strange" or unsteady, sit or lie down immediately.

Discuss syncope and the first-dose effect with your physician before taking Hytrin or other alpha blockers.

When should it be taken? Because Hytrin can produce dizziness and related side effects, it is generally taken before bedtime, at least for the first several days.

Androgen Suppression

The idea behind androgen suppression is to shrink the prostate by depriving it of substances called androgens (male hormones), which encourage it to grow. In other words, take away the growing prostate's food, and let it lose a little weight. Let's take a look at Proscar, the prominent drug in this category.

Proscar (chemical name: finasteride)

Description: Proscar tablets contain 5 mg of finasteride and over a dozen inactive ingredients, including dyes and purified water.

How it works: Proscar is a synthetic compound that cuts back on the amount of DHT (dihydrotestosterone) available to the prostate. It was approved by the FDA for use in the treatment of BPH in June 1992.

DHT comes from testosterone, the male hormone. The conversion from testosterone to DHT is assisted by an enzyme called 5-alpha-reductase in the prostate, the liver, and the skin. DHT is a powerful substance that increases male characteristics—including the tendency of the prostate to develop. Finasteride works by inhibiting the enzyme responsible for the conversion from testosterone to DHT. With less DHT in the prostate, there is less "incentive" for prostatic growth.

Rationale: The idea behind Proscar is an old one. Over one hundred years ago, in 1886, a physician removed both testicles in seventy-nine BPH patients in an attempt to cut off their source of testosterone and relieve their symptoms. Subsequently, in 1940, three men had their testicles removed. Two of these men later had their prostates removed, and there was evidence that their glands had indeed shrunk. Because removing the testicles is a rather extreme method, researchers began looking for drugs that could accomplish the same thing (reducing testosterone), while leaving the testicles intact. The drugs tested were potentially useful, but tended to "feminize" men.

The approach was refined as researchers discovered that the testosterone was converted into DHT in the prostate. Now they could look for ways to attack DHT, rather than testosterone in general. By being more selective, they might be able to reduce the side effects. The search for a new drug got a boost when researchers investigated men with a genetic deficiency of 5-alpha-reductase, who also had lower levels of DHT. These men had urogenital defects at birth, but also had small prostates and did not develop BPH. Was there a way to reproduce the effects of this genetic defect later in life, in normal men?

Meanwhile, scientists in the Caribbean were researching pseudo-hermaphrodites. Hermaphrodites are people with both male and female sexual characteristics, while *pseudo-* (false) hermaphrodites are males who develop male sexual traits in early puberty. The researchers were intrigued by the fact that the prostates of the pseudohermaphrodites did not enlarge as they aged, possibly due to the fact that they lack an enzyme that helps to regulate male hormones. They wondered if there was a way to manipulate enzymes into mimicking the "no prostate growth" effect.

Intended use: The medicine is intended to be used for treating men who have BPH *and* whose BPH has produced symptoms. In other words, you should not be taking the medicine just because your prostate is enlarged. There must be enlargement *and* symptoms before the medicine is indicated.

How well does it work? Although enlarged prostates will shrink in many men, the 1994 *Physicians' Desk Reference* reports that less than 50 percent of the men will enjoy an increase in urinary flow and improvement in BPH symptoms in the course of twelve months of medication. Additionally, you may have to take Proscar for at least six months before learning whether or not you will respond well to the medicine. So far, we can't predict who will be a good candidate for Proscar.

Who should not *take Proscar?*
- Children; it has not been established whether or not Proscar is safe or effective for children.
- Anyone who is hypersensitive to the medicine itself, or to any of the other ingredients in the tablet.
- Proscar is not indicated for women.

Special warning to men: Proscar causes the serum PSA levels to drop, even in patients who have prostate cancer. This means that if you are taking Proscar, and if you have cancer, your PSA test may no longer be a reliable cancer indicator.

Special warning to women: Women who are pregnant, or who may become pregnant, should not take Proscar, should not be exposed to the semen of a man who is taking Proscar, and should avoid handling crushed Proscar tablets. (We don't know how much Proscar a woman can absorb through sexual contact or the handling of crushed Proscar tablets.) The fetus exposed to Proscar may develop abnormalities of the external genitalia.

Side effects: Side effects include impotence, decreased libido, and a smaller volume of ejaculate (less semen).

How much should you take? 5 mg per day is the recommended dose. It may be taken with or without food.

Alpha Blockers versus Finasteride[1]

In a perfect world, I could tell you exactly how well each medication works, what the chances of side effects are, and so on. Unfortunately, the world of medicine and drug testing is not quite perfect. Various studies show different results with the same medications. This happens for various reasons, including the age of the men studied, the way they were selected for the study, the length of the study, the strength of the medications used, and the way the researchers measured the results.

Keep that in mind as you review these U.S. Department of Health and Human Services figures comparing the alpha blockers (such as Hytrin) to the androgen suppressor finasteride (Proscar).

Treatment Outcome	Alpha Blockers	Finasteride
1. Chance for symptom improvement	59–68%	54–78%
2. Degree of symptom improvement	51%	31%
3. Complications	3–43%	14–19%
4. Risk of impotence	NA	2.5–5%
5. Work days lost	3.5	1.5
6. Days in hospital	0	0

*Note: Numbers in the first four items rounded to the nearest 1%.

I don't agree with all of these figures, but they do give us a way to compare the effectiveness and safety of the alpha blockers with those of finasteride.

Combined Therapy

Since the alpha blockers and finasteride attack different aspects of the same problem, would they work better together? Could they relax the smooth muscle of the prostate *and* shrink the gland? The idea makes sense. A large-scale, randomized clinical trial is being conducted by the Department of Veterans Affairs to compare the two drugs in combination against medicines used alone. The combined treatment could prove to be a powerful one-two punch against BPH, but we must wait for the results to see—and to see evidence that the two drugs together don't cause unacceptable side effects.

MEDICINES FOR PROSTATITIS

Today, there is an impressive array of medicines for prostatitis and infections of the urinary tract. Before looking at some of the many drugs, it will be useful to define a few terms:

Aminoglycosides: A class of antibiotics that are related to each other but vary widely in clinical applications. They are all poorly absorbed from the gastrointestinal tract, and are thus most effective when given intramuscularly (i.e., an injection in the buttocks) or intravenously (IV). They can cause serious kidney damage, as well as impaired hearing. Some of the aminoglycosides are streptomycin, neomycin, kanomycin, amikacin, gentamycin, and tobramycin.

Antibiotic: From Greek origins, meaning "against life." Antibiotics are medicines designed to kill bacteria and other microorganisms.

Broad-spectrum: Antibiotics that work against a wide range (spectrum) of organisms, rather than against a specific one. A drawback of the broad-spectrum antibiotics, however, is that they may kill beneficial organisms in addition to the bad ones.

Cephalosporin: Any of several antibiotics that, although able to attack many bacteria, are the drugs of choice for just a few specific bacteria. They are often used as an alternative for patients who are allergic to penicillin.

Chemical name: The name that reflects the general chemical composition of a drug. For example, Proscar's chemical name is 4-azaandrost-1-ene-17-carboxamide, N-(1,1-dimethylethyl)3-oxo-,(5∞, 17ß).

Complicated infections: Infections in which there are other problems. An example is a foot infection complicated by uncontrolled diabetes or septicemia (bacteria in the blood, causing an infection) associated with shock.

Generic name: The general name given to a drug. For example, finasteride is the generic name for the drug popularly known as Proscar.

Penicillins: A large group of antibacterial agents that have a nucleus in common (-6-amino-penicillanic acid). In addition to a natural penicillin, there are semisynthetic penicillins (such as amoxicillin, methacillin, Pen-Vee, ampicillin, oxacillin, and carbenacillin).

Susceptible organisms: Bacteria or other organisms that can be damaged or killed by a particular medicine.

Tetracyclines: A group of closely related, broad-spectrum antibiotics, fairly similar in their effectiveness and toxicity. Some of the tetracyclines are tetracycline, doxycycline, demeclocycline, oxytetracycline, and methacycline.

Trade name: The name given to a medicine by the company that sells it; the popular name by which most people refer to a drug.

Uncomplicated infections: Infections with no associated complicating factors.

Medicines Used for Acute Bacterial Prostatitis

With an understanding of some key drug terms, we now look at how some of the many prostatitis drugs are used.

Carbenicillin indanyl sodium

Trade name: Geocillin

What it is: A semisynthetic penicillin. It kills certain bacteria by interfering with their ability to make cellular walls.

Uses: Because it is primarily excreted in the urine, Geocillin has been shown to be quite effective in the treatment of urinary tract infections.

Adverse effects: Occasional fatal and other serious anaphylactic reactions have occurred with the use of this medicine, and with other penicillins. Additional adverse reactions include nausea, lowering of platelets, lowering of the white cell count, and abnormal liver tests. *Do not take this medication until you and your doctor have discussed your history of reactions or allergies to this or any other drug.*

Ciprofloxacin

Trade name: Cipro

What it is: A synthetic, broad-spectrum antibiotic belonging to the quinolone group.

Uses: Cipro is used to treat infections caused by susceptible strains of organisms found in urinary tract infections, such as *Escherichia coli*, *Klebsiella pneumoniae, Enterobacter cloacae, Proteus mirabilis, Pseudomonas aeruginosa, and Staphylococcus epidermidis*. It is also used for susceptible bacteria in lower respiratory tract and other infections.

Adverse effects: The most frequent adverse effects include abdominal pain, vomiting and diarrhea, nausea, skin rash, headaches, and restlessness. Palpitations, high blood pressure, and angina are also possible. *Do not take this medication until you and your doctor have discussed your history of reactions or allergies to this or any other drug.*

Special Note: Cipro reacts badly with theophylline, a drug often used for asthma (and also found in tea). Serious and fatal reactions have occurred, including cardiac arrest and seizures. Don't take Cipro if you're taking theophylline.

In general, quinolones may stimulate the central nervous system. Thus, it is recommended that those who have cerebral arteriosclerosis and seizures avoid Cipro.

Norfloxacin

Trade name: Noroxin

What it is: A synthetic, broad-spectrum antibacterial agent.

Uses: For treating complicated and uncomplicated infections of the urinary tract caused by *E. coli, Klebsiella pneumoniae, P. mirabilis,* and other bacteria.

Adverse effects: After this antibiotic was marketed, the most common adverse reaction was rashes. Seizures and visual disturbances have also been reported. Other side effects include shortness of breath, anaphylactic reactions, arthritis, muscle pain, and immune system abnormalities. *Do not take this medication until you and your doctor have discussed your history of reactions or allergies to this or any other drug.*

Trimethoprim/sulfamethoxazole

Trade name: Bactrim

What it is: A synthetic antibacterial agent, a combination of trimethoprim and sulfamethoxazole.

Uses: For treating infections of the urinary tract caused by *E. coli, Klebsiella* species, *Enterobacter* species, *Morganella morganii,* and other organisms. Also used for chronic bronchitis, travelers' diarrhea in adults, and *pneumocystis carinii pneumonia.* It is one of the most popular antibiotics prescribed for lower urinary tract infections.

Adverse effects: Do not take Bactrim if you are allergic to sulfas; don't take it if you are also taking diuretics such as HCT (hydrochlorothiazide), blood thinners (such as Coumadin), or anticonvulsant medications. Do not take Bactrim if you have kidney impairment or related problems, if you have a folic acid deficiency (as may be found in older alcoholics), or if you are malnourished. If you develop a skin rash, discontinue the Bactrim. Possible side effects of Bactrim include skin reactions, fulminate liver failure, and problems with the bone marrow. *Do not take this medication until you and your doctor have discussed your history of reactions or allergies to this or any other drug.*

Medicines Used for Chronic Bacterial Prostatitis

With chronic bacterial prostatitis, most men will have symptoms such as lower back pain, urinary urgency, urinary frequency, and painful urination. The prostate may be quite tender upon examination, and there may be clumps of white blood cells in the urine. Clearly, cultures of the urine are necessary to decide which antibiotics are necessary. Following are some of the many antibiotics used for chronic bacterial prostatitis.

Clindamycin

Trade name: Cleocin

What it is: A semisynthetic antibiotic.

Uses: For the treatment of serious infections caused by susceptible anaerobic bacteria (bacteria that grow in the absence of oxygen). It has also been suggested that its use be limited to those patients who are sensitive to penicillin.

Adverse effects: Abdominal pain, nausea, vomiting, diarrhea, rashes and welts, jaundice, abnormal liver-function tests, and decreases in white blood cells are among its side effects. Cleocin has been associated with severe colitis, which may be fatal. *Do not take this medication until you and your doctor have discussed your history of reactions or allergies to this or any other drug.*

Erythromycin

Trade name: E-Mycin (and many others).

What it is: An antibiotic produced by a strain of bacteria (*Streptomyces erythreus*). It belongs to the "macrolide" group of antibiotics.

Uses: For the treatment of infections caused by susceptible bacteria, including those of the upper and lower respiratory tract, skin and soft tissue, and others. It is not considered to be a prostate or urinary tract infection medicine, unless the bacteria are specifically sensitive to erythromycin.

Adverse effects: E-Mycin has been associated with serious colitis, and therefore should be used cautiously in patients with diarrhea, and not at all in patients with impaired liver function. Other adverse effects include nausea, vomiting, abdominal pain, allergic skin reactions, and hypersensitivity reactions. *Do not take this medication until you and your doctor have discussed your history of reactions or allergies to this or any other drug.*

Medicines Used for Urinary Tract Infections

We now turn to some of the medicines used to treat infections of the urinary tract. There really is no such thing as the "best" medicine, because each is designed a little differently. One may be stronger but have more side effects. Or it may work well against three kinds of bacteria but be worthless in the fight against the fourth. Perhaps a certain drug works very well for most people, but you may be one of the few who don't tolerate it well.

There are many antimicrobial drugs used for urinary tract infections in adults, such as ampicillin, cefadoxil, ciprofloxacin, doxycycline, norfloxacin, tetracycline, and trimethoprim. Different doctors use different drugs depending upon their preferences and analyses of specific situations. It is also true that physicians associated with managed care organizations must consider which medicines your insurance will pay for, and prescribe accordingly.

Generally speaking, I like to begin my patients with the older, more established drugs that we know more about. Otherwise, patients are at risk of being guinea pigs who find out that even though the five-year study results were good enough to get the drug approved, something bad happens in the sixth year.

Amikacin

Trade name: Amikin. The generic name is amikacin sulfate.

What it is: A semisynthetic aminoglycoside antibiotic.

Uses: For short-term treatment of certain serious infections caused by microorganisms including *E. coli, Pseudomonas* species, *Klebsiella* species,

Enterobacter species, and others. It may be considered to be the initial therapy in gram-negative infections. Its use is not indicated in uncomplicated episodes of urinary tract infection.

Adverse effects: Loss of hearing, muscle paralysis, blood changes, skin rash, headaches, tremor, nausea, vomiting, and other problems. Amikin, an aminoglycoside, may be dangerous to the kidneys and hearing. It should not be used by women during pregnancy, for it can cause fetal damage. *Do not take this medication until you and your doctor have discussed your history of reactions or allergies to this or any other drug.*

Amoxicillin

Trade name: Augmentin

What it is: An antibiotic made from amoxicillin, which is related to penicillin.

Uses: For infections of the urinary tract caused by ß-lactamase-producing strains of *E. coli, Klebsiella* spp (species), and *Enterobacter* spp. It's also used for lower respiratory tract infections, skin infections, sinusitis, and other problems.

Adverse effects: Penicillin therapy can cause serious, even fatal, hypersensitivity reactions, especially in those with a history of sensitivity to more than one allergen. Other adverse effects include diarrhea, nausea, skin rashes, vomiting, indigestion, anemia, blood changes, anxiety, insomnia, confusion, behavior changes, and dizziness. *Do not take this medication until you and your doctor have discussed your history of reactions or allergies to this or any other drug.*

Ampicillin

Trade name: Omnipen

What it is: A semisynthetic penicillin.

Uses: For genitourinary tract infections caused by *E. coli, P. mirabilis,* enterococci, *Shigella S. typhosa,* and other agents. Also used for gonorrhea, meningitis, and infections of the gastrointestinal tract.

Adverse effects: Nausea, vomiting, pseudomembranous colitis, diarrhea, skin rashes, liver changes, anemia, blood changes, and other problems. *Do not take this medication until you and your doctor have discussed your history of reactions or allergies to this or any other drug.*

Aztreonam

Trade name: Azactam

What it is: A synthetic antibiotic useful against a wide variety of gram-negative aerobic pathogens. It is given intramuscularly (by injection) or intravenously (IV).

Uses: For complicated and uncomplicated urinary tract infections caused by *E. coli, Klebsiella pneumoniae, P. mirabilis, Pseudomonas aeruginosa,* and other agents. Also used in lower respiratory tract infections, gynecologic infections, and other problems.

Adverse effects: Anaphylaxis, blood changes, abdominal cramps, hypotension, hepatitis, jaundice, seizures, confusion, dizziness, altered taste, halitosis, and other problems. *Do not take this medication until you and your doctor have discussed your history of reactions or allergies to this or any other drug.*

Ceftizoxime

Trade name: Cefizox

What it is: A semisynthetic, broad-spectrum, ß-lactamase cephalosporin antibiotic given by injection or IV.

Uses: For treatment of infections caused by susceptible microorganisms such as *E. coli, Pseudomonas,* and *Klebsiella* species.

Adverse effects: Nausea, vomiting, diarrhea, colitis, aplastic anemia, rash, itching, fever, abnormalities in liver function tests, alterations of kidney tests, and, in some patients, seizures. *Do not take this medication until you and your doctor have discussed your history of reactions or allergies to this or any other drug.*

Cefoperazone

Trade name: Cefobid

What it is: A semisynthetic, broad-spectrum, cephalosporin antibiotic for intravenous use.

Uses: For infections of the urinary tract caused by *E. coli* and *Pseudomonas aeruginosa.* Also used for respiratory tract infections, skin infections, peritonitis, and other problems.

Adverse effects: Changes in the blood (such as a decrease in hemoglobin), changes to the immune system (indicated by decreased neutrophils), diarrhea, loose stools, nausea, and vomiting. *Do not take this medication until you and your doctor have discussed your history of reactions or allergies to this or any other drug.*

Cefotaxime

Trade name: Claforan

What it is: A broad-spectrum, cephalosporin antibiotic given by injection or intravenously.

Uses: For infections of the urinary tract produced by *Enterococcus* species, *Staphylococcus epidermidis, Staphylococcus aureus, Citrobacter* species, *Enterobacter* species, *E. coli,* and other agents. Also used for lower respiratory tract infections, gynecological infections, skin infections, bone infections, gonorrhea, and other problems.

Adverse effects: Pain or inflammation at the injection site, rash, fever, colitis, diarrhea, nausea, and vomiting; also blood changes, headaches, and other side effects. *Do not take this medication until you and your doctor have discussed your history of reactions or allergies to this or any other drug.*

Cefoxitin

Trade name: Mefoxin

What it is: A semisynthetic, broad-spectrum antibiotic given intravenously or by injection into the muscle.

Uses: For infections of the urinary tract caused by *E. coli, Klebsiella* species, *P. mirabilis,* and other organisms. Also used for lower respiratory tract infections, gynecological infections, bone and joint infections, and other problems.

Adverse effects: Thrombophlebitis, rash, fever, hypotension, diarrhea, blood changes, and jaundice. *Do not take this medication until you and your doctor have discussed your history of reactions or allergies to this or any other drug. Tell your doctor if you have had any reactions to penicillin, cephalosporins, or if you have any other sensitivities before taking this drug.*

Ceftriaxone

Trade name: Rocephin

What it is: A semisynthetic, broad-spectrum cephalosporin antibiotic.

Uses: Uncomplicated and complicated infections of the urinary tract caused by *E. coli, P. mirabilis, P. vulgaris, Morganella morganii,* or *Klebsiella pneumoniae.*

Adverse effects: Reported side effects include pain or tenderness at the injection site, rash, fever, chills, blood changes, diarrhea, nausea, vomiting, changes in liver and kidney tests, headaches, dizziness, vaginitis, and flushing. *Do not take this medication until you and your doctor have discussed your history of reactions or allergies to this or any other drug.*

Ceftzadime

Trade name: Ceptaz

What it is: A semisynthetic, broad-spectrum antibiotic for intravenous use.

Uses: For complicated and uncomplicated infections of the urinary tract caused by *Psuedomonas aeruginosa, Enterobacter* spp (species), *Proteus* ssp, *Klebsiella* ssp, and *E. coli.*

Adverse effects: Phlebitis, inflammation at the injection site, rash, fever, diarrhea, vomiting, abdominal pain, and other problems. *Do not take this medication until you and your doctor have discussed your history of reactions or allergies to this or any other drug.*

Cefuroxime

Trade name: Ceftin

What it is: A broad-spectrum, cephalosporin antibiotic.

Uses: For infections of the urinary tract produced by *E. coli* and *Klebsiella pneumoniae.* Also used for tonsillitis, lower respiratory tract infection, gonorrhea, and other problems.

Adverse effects: Nausea, vomiting, diarrhea, loose stools, rash, headaches, dizziness, and other problems. *Do not take this medication until you and your doctor have discussed your history of reactions or allergies to this or any other drug.*

Cefadroxil

Trade name: Duricef

What it is: A semisynthetic cephalosporin antibiotic.

Uses: For infections of the urinary tract produced by *E. coli, P. mirabilis,* and *Klebsiella* species.

Adverse effects: Nausea, vomiting, diarrhea, rash, genital pruritus, and blood changes. *Do not take this medication until you and your doctor have discussed your history of reactions or allergies to this or any other drug.*

Doxycycline

Trade name: Vibramycin

What it is: A broad-spectrum antibiotic.

Uses: For uncomplicated urethral infections due to *Chlamydia trachomatis*. Also used for Rocky Mountain spotted fever, typhus fever, respiratory tract infections, and other problems.

Adverse effects: Vibramycin is a member of the tetracycline group of medications. Side effects of tetracyclines include anorexia, nausea, vomiting, diarrhea, hepatotoxicity, rashes, hemolytic anemia, and blood changes. *Do not take this medication until you and your doctor have discussed your history of reactions or allergies to this or any other drug.*

Gentamicin

Trade name: Garamycin

What it is: An antibiotic belonging to the aminoglycoside group.

Uses: For serious urinary tract and other infections.

Adverse effects: Nephrotoxicity, dizziness, vertigo, roaring in the ears, hearing loss, numbness, tingling of the skin, muscle twitching, convulsions, respiratory depression, confusion, depression, visual disturbances, a decrease in appetite, hypotension, and hypertension. *Do not take this medication until you and your doctor have discussed your history of reactions or allergies to this or any other drug.*

Imipenem-cilastatin

Trade name: Primaxin I.V.

What it is: A powerful, broad-spectrum antibacterial for intravenous injection.

Uses: For complicated and uncomplicated infections of the urinary tract caused by *Staphylococcus aureus*, Group D streptococci, *E. coli*, *Klebsiella* spp, *Enterobacter* spp, and other bacteria. Also used for lower respiratory tract infections, bone and joint infections, endocarditis, and other problems.

Adverse effects: Nausea, diarrhea, vomiting, rash, fever, hypotension, seizures, and dizziness were the most frequently reported adverse reactions in clinical trials. *Do not take this medication until you and your doctor have discussed your history of reactions or allergies to this or any other drug.*

Mezlocillin

Trade name: Mezlin

What it is: A semisynthetic, broad-spectrum antibiotic of the penicillin group.

Uses: For urinary tract infections caused by *E. coli, P. mirabilis, Klebsiella* spp, *Enterobacter* spp, and other organisms. Also used for gynecological infections, septicemia, and other problems.

Adverse effects: Skin rashes, changes in taste, diarrhea, blood changes, and convulsive seizures. *Do not take this medication until you and your doctor have discussed your history of reactions or allergies to this or any other drug.*

Netilmicin sulfate

Trade name: Netromycin

What it is: A semisynthetic antibiotic of the aminoglycoside group.

Uses: For complicated urinary tract infections produced by *E. coli, Klebsiella pneumoniae, Pseudomonas aeruginosa, Enterobacter* spp, and other organisms. Also used in septicemia, and in skin and abdominal infections.

Adverse effects: Nephrotoxicity (poisoning of the kidneys, more common among elderly patients, those with a history of kidney impairment, those taking larger than recommended doses, and those taking the drug for longer than recommended periods). Other adverse effects include dizziness, tinnitus, nystagmus, nausea, vomiting, and acute Ménière's syndrome. *Do not take this medication until you and your doctor have discussed your history of reactions or allergies to this or any other drug.*

Nitrofurantoin

Trade name: Macrobid

What it is: An antibacterial agent used specifically for infections of the urinary tract.

Uses: For uncomplicated, acute infections of the urinary tract caused by susceptible *E. coli* or *Staphylococcus saprophyticus* strains.

Adverse effects: Nausea, headaches, flatulence (gas), diarrhea, abdominal pain, constipation, dizziness, drowsiness, pulmonary fibrosis, pancreatitis, peripheral neuropathy, and liver reactions. *Do not take this medication until you and your doctor have discussed your history of reactions or allergies to this or any other drug.*

Piperacillin

Trade name: Pipracil

What it is: A semisynthetic, broad-spectrum penicillin.

Uses: For infections of the urinary tract caused by *E. coli*, enterococci, and other organisms. Also used for lower respiratory tract, skin, and gynecological infections and other problems.

Adverse effects: Although Pipracil is usually tolerated well by patients, adverse effects can include diarrhea, loose stools, vomiting, nausea, liver problems, rashes, headaches, dizziness, fatigue, and blood disturbances. *Do not take this medication until you and your doctor have discussed your history of reactions or allergies to this or any other drug.*

Tetracycline

Trade name: Achromycin

What it is: An antibiotic derived from *Streptomyces aureofaciens*.

Uses: For uncomplicated urethral infections caused by *Chlamydia trachomatis* and many other infections.

Adverse effects: Nausea, vomiting, diarrhea, pancreatitis, esophagitis, skin rashes, and blood changes. *Do not take this medication until you and your doctor have discussed your history of reactions or allergies to this or any other drug.*

Tobramycin

Trade name: Nebcin

What it is: An antibiotic.

Uses: For complicated and recurrent infections of the urinary tract produced by *P. aeruginosa, Proteus* spp, *E. coli, Klebsiella* spp, *Enterobacter* spp, *Serratia* spp, *S. aureus, Providencia* spp, and *Citrobacter* spp.

Adverse effects: Dizziness, vertigo, a roaring sound in the ears, loss of hearing, damage to the kidneys, and blood changes. Your doctor should watch you closely if he gives you Nebcin (or other aminoglycosides). Nebcin may prompt nephrotoxicity, neurotoxicity, and ototoxicity. *Do not take this medication until you and your doctor have discussed your history of reactions or allergies to this or any other drug.*

Although these are not the only medicines used for BPH and prostatitis, they are representative, including benefits and risks.

QUESTIONS TO ASK BEFORE TAKING *ANY* MEDICINE

Make sure both you and your doctor understand the indications that suggest the need for a particular medicine, as well as its toxicities and expected course. It will be mutually helpful to discuss the pros and cons of the suggested drug, as well as the alternative treatments. Finally, before taking any medicine, talk to your doctor as follows:

1. Ask why you need the drug.
2. Explain which drugs, nutritional supplements, and other substances you are currently taking.
3. Tell if you have ever had *any* adverse reactions, sensitivity reactions, or allergies to *any* drug, or if you have any allergies to any other substances.
4. Ask when the drug should be taken, how many times a day, and whether it should be taken with food or water.
5. Ask the doctor to review *all* of the side effects with you.
6. Ask for descriptions of the early signs of side effects.
7. Ask if another, less powerful, medicine could be used instead.
8. Ask how you will know if the drug is working.
9. Ask which drug the doctor would take, or would give to his or her family, to treat the same problem.

10. Ask if a generic version of the drug, which is usually less expensive, is available.
11. Ask if there are any nondrug treatments available.

Remember: Every single drug has side effects, and many doctors prescribe drugs all too easily. There is no law saying that you must blindly take medicine that is prescribed. Ask your physician—and ask yourself—if you really need the drug, and if the benefits outweigh the risks.

5

Surgeries for the Prostate

While there are many effective, less invasive treatments, surgery is called for in many cases. This chapter reviews the most common prostate surgeries for both cancer and BPH, then briefly discusses anesthesia. Reading this won't make you a surgeon, but it will give you enough information to discuss these surgeries in an informed way with your doctor.

WHAT TO ASK BEFORE AGREEING TO SURGERY

Many individuals are afraid of surgery. I consider any surgery performed on me, no matter how small, to be very major. Surgery can do wonders, but it's definitely not for everyone. That's why everyone should carefully consider *all* of the alternatives to surgery, and weigh the potential benefits against the drawbacks (I advise all of my patients to do so).

Before agreeing to undergo surgery, ask your doctor(s) as many questions as possible. Here are twenty-three questions that will more than get the discussion started:

1. Why are you recommending this surgery?
2. What are the goals of this surgery? What do you hope to accomplish?
3. How will we know if the surgery has worked? What signs of improvement can I expect to see, and when?
4. Please describe the surgery. What happens, where would I be cut, and what is removed.
5. What are the side effects? What do you do to keep the side effects to a minimum, or to deal with them after surgery?

72

6. What alternative surgeries or treatments are available? Why are you recommending this surgery instead of any of the alternatives?

7. What would happen if I had no surgery at all? Is "watchful waiting" a viable option for me?

8. How long will I be in the hospital?

9. How many tubes will be sticking out of my body when I wake up? What are they for? How long will they be in place?

10. How soon will I be able to return to work following the surgery?

11. Will any of my activities be restricted following the surgery? Which ones, and for how long?

12. Will I be taking postoperative medications? If so, which ones, why, for how long, and what side effects do they have?

13. Impotence is a potential side effect of prostate surgery. What percentage of these surgeries cause impotence? What treatments will be available to me should I become impotent?

14. Incontinence is a potential side effect of prostate surgery. What percentage of these surgeries cause incontinence? What treatments will be available to me should I become incontinent?

15. Will you give me the names of some patients who have undergone this surgery, so I can speak to them?

16. How extensive is the patient education information that you provide on this surgery? Can you recommend any articles or books for me to read?

17. How many of these surgeries have you performed? How many of your patients having this surgery have returned to full activity? How many have died?

18. What kind of anesthesia will be used? Why that kind? Are there possible or probable side effects? Who will perform the anesthesiology? Will I meet the anesthesiologist prior to surgery?

19. At which hospital will the surgery be performed? How many of these surgeries are done at this hospital per year?

20. How much does the surgery cost? What is your fee, the fee for the assistant surgeon(s), the fee for the anesthesiologist, the hospital fee? What are fees for postoperative care, and any additional costs?

21. Will your office staff help me to find out if my insurance covers this surgery? Will your office staff help me to fill out the insurance forms?

22. Whom do you recommend that I see for a second opinion?

Don't be afraid to ask your doctor questions! It's your body, you are paying the money, you are the boss, and you can ask all the questions you like. As previously suggested, if the doctor doesn't want to answer your questions, it's time to look for one who will.

You can assist your doctor in these early discussions by reading up on your disease, and by preparing your questions in advance. Some patients mail their questions to the physician's office before their visit, providing time for review before the critical consultation.

Now let's look at the major prostate surgeries, beginning with the often-performed radical prostatectomy.

RADICAL PROSTATECTOMY

Radical prostatectomy is the surgical removal of the prostate. Also known as an "open prostatectomy" or a "radical," it is a major surgery in which the patient's body is cut open and the entire prostate is removed. It's a very popular surgery. According to a report in the *Journal of the American Medical Association,* "almost as many radical prostatectomies were performed [on Medicare patients] in 1990 as were performed in 1984 through 1987 combined."[1]

The radical prostatectomy is generally performed on prostate cancer patients in order to remove the entire cancerous growth from the body. The idea is a sound one: Get the cancer out of the body before it spreads. That is the result, however, only if the cancer is truly confined to the prostate, and if the surgery eliminates every last cancer cell.

If the cancer has spread beyond the prostate—even a little bit beyond—removing the prostate will not halt the disease. And if just a few cells escape the surgeon's knife, the cancer can grow back to full size and strength. *Radical prostatectomy makes sense only if the surgeon can excise all of the cancer.*

The two approaches to radical prostatectomy are *retropubic radical prostatectomy,* in which the surgeon cuts into your lower abdomen to get to the prostate, and *perineal radical prostatectomy,* in which the surgeon cuts into the area between your scrotum and anus to get to the prostate. The procedure detailed here is the retropubic radical prostatectomy—the more frequently performed of the two.

Before Your Prostatectomy

Your doctor will perform several, or perhaps many, of the tests described in Chapter 3 to assist in planning the surgery. These tests may be frightening, uncomfortable, or outright painful. Ask why each test is necessary, and if there are alternatives to any of the tests that you fear may be unendurable. And feel free to ask your doctor or the technician performing the test all about it. Many patients feel better knowing what is going to happen, what is actually happening, why the machine is making noise, and what the odd lines on the screen mean.

You may also be asked to make an autologous blood donation—a donation to yourself. Blood is drawn from your arm at intervals and stored for up to a month before the surgery, in case you may need blood replacement during the operation or afterward. Using your own blood eliminates the chances of acquiring hepatitis, HIV, or other diseases; it is also felt that restoring one's own blood is more immediately therapeutic during the surgery.

You may be asked to take iron supplements for your blood, and to stop taking aspirin and any medicines that contain aspirin for a week or two before your surgery. Aspirin can cause increased bleeding, so your doctor will want to make sure it's out of your system before performing surgery.

Finally, you'll be asked to undergo an examination by your personal physician or another internist. The general physical examination verifies that you are healthy enough to have surgery.

A Typical "Radical"

In a typical radical retropubic prostatectomy with lymph node dissection, the surgeon cuts into the man's lower abdomen. The cut runs from the belly button down approximately six inches toward the pubic bone.

The muscles layered underneath the skin in the abdomen are the rectus muscles, those you feel working when you are doing sit-ups. These muscles are not cut. Instead, the surgeon slits the fascia that holds muscle bands together, and pulls the muscles to the side, anchoring them in place out of the way.

Now the doctor is into the area where the bladder and the prostate sit. Since the lymph nodes are going to be examined, the doctor removes the nodes that run along the blood vessels, perhaps one to three inches away from the side of the prostate. These are the lymph nodes to which the prostate cancer is likely to have spread first, if it has spread at all. The nodes themselves are small, perhaps the size of a fingernail. Once removed, the nodes are sent to the laboratory for immediate analysis. If the nodes are cancerous, the surgeon may close the patient up without removing the prostate, feeling that there is no point to removing the prostate since the cancer has already spread. If, however, the laboratory should find that there is no cancer in the lymph nodes, the surgeon will proceed.

Even though the surgeon has entered the area holding the bladder and prostate, it's hard to tell which is which at a glance because most of the tissue inside the body is covered with a thin layer of fat, giving it a yellowish look. With a probing finger, however, the surgeon can feel that the bladder is soft and flexible, like an empty balloon with a thick wall. Together, the bladder and prostate look something like an upside-down pear, with the fat part being the bladder, and the skinny part being the prostate.

Now that the prostate has been located, it must be removed. The surgeon begins by cutting away some of the tissue attached to the sides of the prostate, making it more mobile, and allowing closer access to the bottom of the prostate (which is attached to the urethra).

It gets tricky now, because a bundle of veins called the dorsal venous complex runs across the top of the urethra. The veins must be carefully clamped off before being cut to prevent bleeding. When the veins have been clamped and cut, the surgeon can cut the urethra free from the prostate.

The surgeon continues cutting around the prostate to release it. If this is a nerve-sparing surgery, the doctor will be very careful as the prostate is cut free from surrounding tissue, because nerves vital to the penis run very close to the prostate. In fact, the nerves are sort of attached to the prostate, so they must be peeled away with care. Instead of cutting widely around the prostate and severing these nerves, the surgeon must cut very close to the prostate to avoid damaging them.

The surgeon continues cutting the prostate free, working up toward the bladder. The seminal vesicles are cut out with the prostate, and the vas deferens are tied off and left in place.

Now the prostate is free, except for where it is attached to the bladder above. The surgeon cuts into the bladder, essentially cutting a hole in the bottom of the bladder to release the prostate. (The "bottom" of the bladder is the "top" of the prostate, so it's impossible to cut out the prostate without cutting such a hole.) The surgeon can now remove the prostate from the patient's body.

The surgeon inspects the bladder to make sure there is no damage other than the hole in the bottom, which is about the size of a quarter. Then stitches are used to shrink the quarter-sized hole down to about the size of a dime. Finally, the bladder is pulled down to the urethra, and the two are stitched together.

SURGERIES FOR THE PROSTATE

The surgery is complete. The surgeon cleans the area by irrigating it with fluid, and closes up any small blood vessels that might still be bleeding. Because the seam between the bladder and the urethra is new and not tightly closed, fluid will leak out into the surrounding tissues during the first day or two after surgery, so the doctor lays a tube in the area. The tube comes out of the body through a small slit in the skin a little bit to the side of the original incision, and drains into a small suction device that may be taped to the patient's abdomen.

The patient is ready to be closed up. The muscle bands are loosely brought together with stitches, and the fascia layer is carefully stitched together. (Remember, the fascia holding muscle bands together was cut, but the muscles themselves were not.) The fat layer is generally left alone, because fat does not hold stitches well. Finally, the skin is sutured or "stapled" together.

Assuming that all goes well, the entire procedure takes two and a half to three hours from the time the first incision is made until the patient is ready to be wheeled out of surgery. Patients are generally able to go home three to five days after surgery.

How Is the Decision to Have Surgery Made?

Most people undoubtedly think that doctors have very firm, objective criteria for selecting who should have surgery, and which surgery is most appropriate. The truth is, however, that we don't have formulas or computer programs that tell us which surgery is best for which patient. Whether or not you have surgery and which surgery will be recommended for you depends upon many factors, including who your doctor is, where he or she trained, and your surgeon's personal preferences.

A study reported in the May 26, 1993, issue of the Journal of the American Medical Association found that the part of the country in which you happen to live plays a large role in determining whether you will have a radical prostatectomy.[2] The authors studied Medicare patients from 1984 through 1990 and found that the rate of radical prostatectomy varied widely from state to state. For example, between 1988 and 1990, there were 429 radical prostatectomies for every 100,000 male Medicare beneficiaries in Alaska, the number one state for the surgery, compared to only 20 in Rhode Island.

What Happens after the Radical Prostatectomy?

You will likely wake up to find a number of tubes in your body, such as:

IVs (intravenous lines)

One or more of these small tubes will be attached by a needle to your arm, and to a bottle suspended above your bed. The IVs are used to deliver nourishment, medicines, and blood (if necessary).

Patient-controlled analgesia tube

This IV tube is also connected to your arm by a needle, and leads to a container of pain medicine on the other end. A conveniently placed control device allows you to regulate the amount of pain medicine you get.

Suction drain

This tube, which seems to be growing right out of your lower abdomen, drains fluids and blood from the surgical site. Getting rid of the excess fluids helps reduce the risk of infection. Typically, the drainage tube will be removed within a few days of surgery, while you are still in the hospital. The doctor usually cuts the stitch that holds the tube in place, and gently pulls it out. You may feel a little burning sensation as the tube comes out, leaving behind it a small hole that will be covered with some gauze. (Stitches are not generally required.)

A catheter

This is a special tube that comes out of the penis and drains into a collecting bag that is hung on the bed. With the catheter in place, urine coming into the bladder from the kidneys automatically drains out into the bag. If the man has had a nerve-sparing operation, and if he happens to get an erection, there should be no problem with the catheter.

When you want to walk around, you can connect the catheter to a smaller bag that straps on to your thigh. You can wear either a hospital gown or a loose pair of pants over the collecting bag. If all goes well, there should be no spillage, no smell, and no sloshing sounds coming from the bag.

The smaller "home" bags come in half-liter and one-liter sizes and usually have to be emptied every four hours or so. To empty them, you simply walk up to the toilet as if you were going to urinate, hold the bag over the toilet, open a valve at the bottom of the bag, and let it drain. The catheter and bags require no special care, although if the catheter gets dry, it may irritate the tip of the penis. KY jelly or other lubricants help. You should not use Vaseline, however, because that can dissolve the catheter. Soap and water are very helpful for keeping everything clean.

You may also be given oral medications such as pain medicines, antibiotics, iron pills for your blood, a stool softener to keep you from straining when defecating, and a laxative.

When You Leave the Hospital . . .

You will probably be given two different kinds of collecting bags to attach to the catheter that is still draining urine from your bladder. We previously mentioned the smaller "leg bag" that attaches to your thigh, hiding under your pants. The larger bag is used for overnight and for when you know you'll be managing the catheter at home for a while.

You may see some small clots of blood in your urine bag, or notice that the urine is pinkish (from blood leaking into the urine). This is normal, but pay attention to how much there is, and call your doctor if the bleeding is heavy, or if it continues.

The catheter in the bladder can cause pain for which bladder antispasmodic medicines are helpful. The catheter is usually removed when the patient returns to the doctor's office in about two weeks for a follow-up visit. The doctor simply deflates the balloon that has been holding the catheter in place by draining the water out of the balloon through a port at the end of the catheter. With the balloon flattened, the catheter comes out easily. You may want to bring a pad with you when the catheter is removed, in case you have trouble with incontinence. There are several kinds of these pads available commercially.

You will also be given a plethora of instructions. These vary from doctor to doctor, but will likely include admonitions to:

- Fill your prescriptions.
- Stay out of the bathtub, hot tubs, and swimming pools. Showers are permitted.
- Perform gentle exercise, such as simple walking, as much as possible. Avoid strenuous exercise or sports for several weeks to several months. Practice any prescribed exercises.
- Do not drive or operate heavy or dangerous machinery for up to four to six weeks after surgery, or until permitted by your doctor.
- Pay attention to what is happening to you, so that you can provide accurate reports to the doctor at the appointed time.

Expect to have mild to total urinary incontinence after your radical prostatectomy. How long one suffers from incontinence, and to what degree, varies from man to man. Some men are urinating normally almost immediately, and some within a few weeks; others never recover full continence.

Benefits of a Radical Prostatectomy

If the cancer is restricted to the prostate, and *if* the surgery removes every single cancerous cell, the surgery has been a big success. Unfortunately, in many, many cases at least some of the cancer is left behind and comes back to threaten the patient in later years. Even if the cancer recurs, however, the surgery can still be considered successful if the cancer is held at bay for a significant period of time, and if the patient considers the trade-off between delaying the cancer and suffering the side effects to be worthwhile.

Again, assuming all goes very well, you won't have to worry about the cancer again, and you won't have to take any medicines or hormones for the prostate cancer for the rest of your life.

Drawbacks of a Radical Prostatectomy

The primary complications of a radical prostatectomy are incontinence and impotence. The statistics vary widely as to how many men will wind up with urinary and sexual difficulties, and for how long. A Johns Hopkins study, in which men were operated on in the most ideal conditions, found that 50 percent were incontinent three months after the operations and 8 percent were still incontinent after twenty-four months. The study determined that up to 50 percent will suffer from long-term impotence, depending on their age and the type of surgery.

Less common, but more threatening, is the very small but real possibility (generally less than 1 percent) of death that goes along with *any* surgery.

Who Should Have a Radical and
Who Should Avoid It

Although surgeons are operating on increasing numbers of prostate cancer patients, including older men, I believe that the radical prostatectomy should only be performed if:

- the doctor can confidently say that the cancer is truly confined to the prostate, and
- the patient is young and healthy enough that he is very likely to live another ten or more years, and
- the patient understands that, even with a nerve-sparing operation, he may wind up impotent, and
- the patient realizes that he may end up wearing diapers for an extended period of time, and
- the patient has consulted with other physicians who have explained the relative benefits of other treatments, including hormonal therapy, radiation, and alternative therapies.

Although the open, or radical, prostatectomy is considered the "gold standard" of prostate cancer surgery, many surgeries and surgical procedures for cancer and BPH have been devised in recent years. Let's take a look at the new approaches, beginning with cryosurgery.

CRYOSURGERY

Cryosurgery is the "ice cube" surgery, an attempt to destroy cancer cells by literally freezing them to death. The approach was originally used for prostate cancer back in the 1960s, but the results were not very encouraging. The technique has been revived in recent years, with new technology providing more favorable results. Although more and more medical centers across the country are offering cryosurgery, it is still considered experimental by most urologists.

Cryosurgery is a new procedure—too new for us to know how well it works in the long run, and whether it will become a standard treatment for prostate cancer in the future. The Food and Drug Administration has approved cryosurgery for use in humans, but it has not been endorsed by the major medical organizations.[3]

How It Works

The cells of the body (and the molecules, enzymes, and other substances within them) are designed to work within a limited temperature range. As the temperature falls, the molecular processes within a cell slow down, and may eventually halt altogether. Freezing the cells can cause ionic imbalance, disruption of the acid-base balance, energy deprivation, denaturation of proteins, disruption of membranes, shearing (ripping) of the cell wall, and other stresses leading to cellular death. Freezing can also cause the cells to become dehydrated by drawing water out of them and into the intracellular spaces, where it becomes ice. In addition, blood vessels supplying the area are destroyed.

The general idea is simple: Guided by ultrasound, probes are inserted into the patient's body through small cuts in the perineal area (between the scrotum and the rectum). When everything is in place, liquid nitrogen is circulated through the probes, and the entire prostate gland is frozen. A catheter filled with warm water is placed in the urethra to make sure that the urethra is not frozen and thereby injured.

A Typical Cryosurgery

The patient is placed in the lithotomy position on the operating table (on his back, with his legs spread). He is given general anesthesia, and an ultrasound probe is placed in the rectum.

The surgery is relatively new and procedures have not been standardized, so individual surgeons may have their own specific techniques. Generally, the surgeon begins by inserting a superpubic catheter (a tube running from outside of the body through the belly into the bladder). Using a needle and a guide wire, the surgeon passes the catheter through a small incision into the bladder, then fills the bladder with water. The patient's body temperature warms the water up, and the warm water protects the bladder from injury during the freezing process. This catheter is also used to drain the bladder after the surgery, as internal swelling can make it difficult to urinate normally.

Next the freezing probes are painstakingly put into place. Using a stereotactic guide, up to five needles are inserted into the patient's perineal area. The surgeon watches the ultrasound monitor as, one by one, the needles are slid into the prostate. Then the center of each needle, called the trochar, is pulled out, and a guide wire is slid up through the now-hollow needle. The doctor watches to make sure the guide wire is properly placed. Then the needle is pulled out, leaving only the very thin guide wire in place. This is done until the proper number of wires are embedded in the prostate.

Then the surgeon makes stab wounds in the skin, one exactly where each guide wire passes into the patient. This is done in order to make the openings a little larger so the surgeon can slide a larger piece of instrumentation called a dilator over the guide wires. When the dilators are in place, all the dilators and guide wires are pulled out, leaving only the outer "wrappings" of the dilators, called sheaths, in place in the prostate. The probes that do the actual freezing are then slid into place through the sheaths.

There's a lot of sliding in and out, as needles, guide wires, and dilators are carefully placed. The end result is the strategic placement of up to five probes.

Now the freezing begins. Liquid nitrogen is pumped into the probes. An iceball begins to form around the tip of each probe as prostatic tissue is frozen. The surgeon has carefully placed the probes so that there will be no "holes" in the freezing; eventually the entire prostate will be frozen, leaving no "warm" spots where the cancer might survive. The individual ice balls soon coalesce, turning the entire prostate into one large iceball. If the prostate is very large, it may have to be frozen in sections. The entire surgery takes two to three hours.

When the prostate and surrounding tissue have been completely frozen, the probes are removed. Each small incision is closed up with a stitch or two. When you wake up, you'll notice the suprapubic tube popping out of your abdomen, just below the navel. This tube (used to help drain urine from the bladder) will remain in place for a week or two, depending upon how long it takes until you can urinate normally. The tube connects to a bag attached to your leg. There's a stopcock valve on the tube, so patients can close off the tube and try urinating by themselves.

You may also notice several small puncture wounds behind your scrotum, and you will likely use a "hemorrhoid doughnut" (an inflated plastic ring) when sitting down for a week or two after the surgery.

Benefits of Cryosurgery

Cryosurgery is easier on patients than the radical prostatectomy. There tends to be less blood loss, so transfusions are rarely required. Also, some doctors report that there is less incontinence with cryosurgery than there is with radical prostatectomy. There's also less postoperative pain because the doctor is not making a major incision in the patient's body. The patient can be out of the hospital in a day or two, and back performing most normal activities within a week or so. Because it is less physically demanding, cryosurgery may be performed on some patients who are not healthy enough to withstand the rigors of an open prostatectomy.

Another advantage of cryosurgery is that it can be repeated should the first surgery fail to completely remove the cancer. The costs for cryosurgery are typically about half of those for radical prostatectomy.

Drawbacks to Cryosurgery

Although it is a "smaller" surgery than a radical prostatectomy, cryosurgery still presents all the risks of surgery, including adverse reactions to anesthesia, blood loss, infections, and surgical errors. Incontinence is a significant side effect. Damage to the urethra is possible, leading to "sloughing" of the urethra: Bits of urethral tissue will break off and flow out with the urine. Thus, if the urethra is sloughing, the man will notice particulate matter (bits of flesh) in his urine. His stream may be good then bad, and there may be dribbling. Fifteen percent of patients may have significant sloughing, and all patients who have had previous prostate surgery can expect sloughing. The sloughing can occur for as long as one month after the cryosurgery. The surgery may also result in fistulas (unwanted "tunnels") between the urethra and the rectum, which allow urine to flow into the rectum as well as stool to pass into the urethra or bladder.

Unless they have "nerve-sparing" cryosurgery, all patients will be impotent. This happens because areas beyond the prostate are frozen and destroyed, including the nerves to the penis. Unfortunately, the nerve-sparing procedure is appropriate only for a relatively small number of men. (You will remember that the nerves running to the penis are very close to the prostate, and difficult to spare during surgery or cryosurgery. Even if they could save the nerves, most surgeons prefer to take them out or freeze them, preferring a thorough approach rather than risk leaving behind a few unnoticed cancer cells.)

Shown on the following two pages is a typical "Cryosurgery Consent Form" that patients will be asked to sign before having the surgery. Studying a well-designed consent form that spells out all the possible dangers can be very educational for a man considering the surgery. (This particular form was provided by Douglas Chinn, M.D., of the Alhambra Hospital Cryosurgical Center of Southern California.) Although I do not necessarily agree with all of the side-effect statistics, I find that this information-packed form effectively spells out the potential risks and side effects.

Cryosurgery Consent Form

A urethral warmer is necessary for the operation. It is not FDA approved. Thermocouples to monitor freezing temperatures will also be used. These are also not FDA approved.

Medicare and some private insurance companies will not pay for this procedure.

We do not have long-term follow-up (5 to 10 years) with cryosurgery to evaluate recurrence of the cancer.

More than one cryosurgical treatment may be necessary if future biopsies reveal inadequate freezing of certain areas. This will depend upon the size and location of the cancer. There is currently an 80 percent negative biopsy rate, post-cryosurgery, for stage-B disease.

All patients who have cryosurgical ablation of the prostate will have to have repeat ultrasound-guided biopsies of the prostate at three months, twelve months, and twenty-four months. We may also rebiopsy at some other time interval, depending upon the circumstances.

Following is a summary of the risks and complications of cryosurgery:

1. Anesthesia: Death, myocardial infarction, cerebrovascular accident, and pulmonary embolism can occur with any operation.

2. Bleeding: As with any surgery, bleeding can occur. Rarely is a transfusion necessary.

3. Infection: Urinary tract infection can occur in any urologic operation. Abscess formation, requiring surgical drainage, can occur with any operation.

(continued)

(Continued from previous page)

4. Impotence: In cryosurgery, it is very important to freeze the nerves; as a result impotence SHOULD OCCUR.

5. Incontinence: Currently, there is a 1 percent incontinence with surgery, and 3 to 10 percent with radical prostatectomy. Many patients do have urge and stress incontinence up to three months afterward.

6. Urethral stricture: Occurrence is 1 to 3 percent with either cryosurgery or radical prostatectomy.

7. Bladder neck contracture: Occurrence is 1 to 3 percent with radical prostatectomy, and probably with cryosurgery.

8. Urethral-rectal fistula: Can occur with cryosurgery. Surgical repair will be required, perhaps multiple operations, including a colostomy.

9. Equipment failure: If this occurs, the procedure will be aborted, and repeated at a later date.

10. Hypothermia:[4] This could occur.

11. Bladder or urethral injury: If this occurs, open surgery repair will be required at a later date.

12. Urethral sloughing:[5] This has occurred in 15 percent of cases with the urethral warmer.

13. Urgency and frequency: Fifty percent of patients have urgency and frequency of urination up to three months after the procedure.

14. Urinary retention: Some patients (especially those with preexisting obstruction) may have retention problems for up to eight weeks. In those with preexisting problems, a TURP (transurethral resection of the prostate) may later be required.

Who Should Have Cryosurgery and Who Should Avoid It

Proponents of cryosurgery suggest that any man who is a candidate for a radical prostatectomy or radiation is also a candidate for cryosurgery. Men who are not healthy enough for a radical prostatectomy or radiation, or who are reluctant to undergo surgery or radiation, may wish to discuss cryosurgery with their physicians. Cryosurgery has also been used on men who have had a "failed" surgery or radiation therapy ("failed" meaning that the surgery or radiation did not work). However, there is a higher risk of complications and less chance of success if you've already failed radiation.

Men with bleeding problems such as hemophilia who are not candidates for surgery *should not have cryosurgery,* either. Also, men with prostates larger than approximately 50 grams in weight are usually not good candidates for the "freeze." Some doctors put their patients with large prostates on Lupron or other medications for several months, in an attempt to shrink the gland down to a freezable size. Other doctors will perform two cryosurgeries on the patient with the large prostate. The first surgery freezes the outside parts of the prostate, and, a few months later, a second surgery chills the inner parts of the gland. Some prostates cannot be totally frozen because of odd growth patterns (such as BPH growth in which part of the prostate pushes up into the bladder). Patients with odd-shaped prostates may require a TURP (transurethral resection of the prostate) after the cryosurgery, in order to scrape out the odd-shaped part of the prostate that could not be frozen. (This part of the prostate usually does not contain cancer.)

How Does One Feel after Cryosurgery?

The excerpts from the "Prostate Cryosurgery Postoperative Instructions" sheet that appear on the following page give you an idea of what one can expect after cryosurgery. The postoperative information sheet was provided by doctors at the University of California, San Diego, Medical Center for their patients who have undergone prostatic cryosurgery. *This information is presented for educational purposes only. It is not to be construed as instructions for your surgery. Please consult your physician for your instructions, should you undergo surgery.*

After Your Cryosurgery

ACTIVITY

1. You will have swelling and bruising of your penis and scrotum.
2. It is OK to use ice packs to the scrotum and behind the scrotum, 2 hours at a time with a ½-hour break. The ice packs will help minimize the swelling. Use the ice packs for 2 to 3 days. Some men may require a longer period. Wearing a jockstrap also helps.
3. Keeping off your feet will also help decrease the swelling. You may find that during the day when you are sitting up or walking around, the swelling will increase. You may get up to do minimal daily routines, but staying off your feet the rest of the time, for 2 to 3 days, will help decrease the swelling. Some men may require a longer period of rest.
4. You may shower the second day after surgery.

CARE OF THE SUPRAPUBIC CATHETER

1. After 5 to 7 days, clamp your suprapubic catheter: Attempt to urinate normally without straining; measure the amount voided. After urinating, or if you are unable to urinate, open the suprapubic tube, drain, and measure the amount in a measuring cup and record the amount.
2. Suprapubic tube dressing: Take two 4×4 gauze dressings, place one above and one below the tube, and secure them with tape. Change the dressing daily after cleaning the area around the tube with hydrogen peroxide or soap and water.
3. Numbness at the tip of the penis may be experienced for a period of time after surgery.

Like other standard treatments for prostate cancer, cryosurgery cannot cure cancer that has spread too far beyond the prostate.

Please note that we do not have good, long-term data on the effectiveness of cryosurgery because it is relatively new. Initial results show promise, but it is too early to say that cryosurgery is definitely superior to other approaches over the long run.

TRANSURETHRAL RESECTION OF THE PROSTATE (TURP)

Transurethral resection of the prostate (TURP) is the first of the surgeries for BPH to be discussed. During a TURP, which some call the "Roto-Rooter" surgery, parts of the prostate are removed by an instrument inserted in the urethra at the opening of the penis. Urologists are performing 400,000 TURPs a year, making it one of the most "popular" surgeries in the United States.

TURP is performed to assist in treatment of urinary problems caused by overgrowth of the prostate. As the prostate enlarges, it can squeeze down on the prostatic urethra, causing slowing of the urinary stream, frequency of urination, straining while urinating, feeling that the bladder is not completely emptied, dribbling after voiding, incontinence, and an increased susceptibility to urinary tract infections.

A Typical TURP

A TURP is performed under general or spinal anesthetic. The entire procedure is performed through a resectoscope, as pictured in Figure 5.1, and generally takes an hour or less. There's a lens at the end of the scope, allowing the doctor to see inside the man's body.

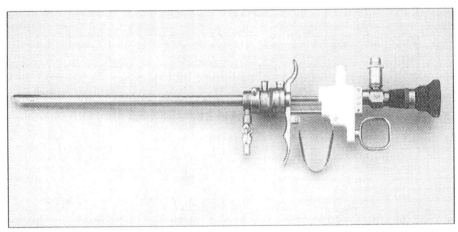

FIGURE 5.1 Resectoscope. *Photo courtesy of Olympus America Inc.*

The scope is pushed into the tip of the penis and up the urethra. (A brace to hold the penis is not necessary.) When the scope reaches the prostate, the doctor can see which tissue is overgrown. As the scope moves up the urethra, it is like walking through a wide-open tunnel and suddenly seeing a collapsed portion. The collapsed part is the overgrown prostatic tissue. Instead of being a wide-open tunnel, the prostatic urethra looks more like a narrow hallway.

The resectoscope has various ports, allowing the doctor to continuously irrigate (wash out) the surgical site while working. The surgery is done with a wire loop, which is advanced and retracted with a lever. The surgeon touches the loop to the selected tissue, then slides the loop back, shaving off slivers of the prostate. A current running through the loop allows it to slice easily through tissue. The doctor can change the current to a coagulating one, a current that will cauterize the tissue to help stop the bleeding.

Essentially, the doctor shaves away the narrowed walls from the inside during a TURP. As the overgrown tissue is eliminated, the narrowed hallway becomes a wide-open tunnel again. Actually, the doctor shaves away healthy prostatic tissue as well, creating an opening much wider than will be necessary. This is because the channel will likely narrow somewhat after the surgery, so it has to be made wider than it will eventually need to be.

The doctor has to be careful when cutting near the areas where the prostate and the urethra meet, and is alert to avoid cutting through the wall of the prostatic capsule (the outer "skin" of the prostate). The doctor can actually see where the bladder begins: The prostate area looks like a narrowed hallway, while the opening of the bladder is rounded.

When surgery is completed, the doctor irrigates the bladder to suck out the many chips of prostate tissue that have floated up into the bladder. When the bladder is clear and all bleeding has been cauterized, the scope is removed and a catheter is put in place. This is a special "three-way" catheter with extra channels to allow for irrigation. The circulating water flushes out blood that will continue to ooze from the prostatic tissue.

After the TURP

Following the procedure, you will have a catheter coming from your penis and an IV tube attached to your arm. The IV generally comes out as soon as you start to drink fluids, which is usually that same evening. The catheter remains in place for a day or so. If all goes well, the catheter is removed the next morning, you will urinate within an hour or two, and then go home. The doctor will want to make sure you can urinate before releasing you.

Expect your urine to be bloody for a few weeks or even a month following a TURP. At a minimum, your urine will be tinged with blood. If there are blood clots in the urine, or the urine seems to be too bloody, call your doctor right away.

Benefits of a TURP

As a surgery for BPH, the TURP is less severe than is the radical prostatectomy. The patient is up and around sooner, with a shorter hospital stay and possibly less medication. The symptoms of BPH often clear up quickly with a TURP.

Drawbacks to a TURP

Although TURP is a smaller surgery than a radical prostatectomy, it is still a surgery, with all the implied risks. There is also the possibility of what is known as "TURP syndrome," a problem that strikes a very small number of men undergoing TURP. The syndrome hits when fluid used to irrigate the area during the surgery is absorbed by the body, leading to nausea and vomiting, mental confusion, hypertension, visual disturbances, and problems with the heartbeat. The larger the prostate and the longer the surgery, the greater the risk of TURP syndrome.

There are also possible sexual side effects. The prostate will still make prostatic fluid following a TURP, but most patients will suffer from "retrograde ejaculation." Because the surgery has created such a wide channel, the prostate won't be able to "close up" the channel and squirt out the ejaculatory fluid. As a result, most of the fluid will run backward (retrograde), up to the bladder instead of down through the urethra. Retrograde ejaculation is painless, but, of course, can make a man infertile. Impotence is also a possible complication. Although some studies have suggested that as many as 13 percent of men undergoing TURP can wind up at least temporarily impotent, the numbers are subject to debate.

Who Should Have a TURP and Who Should Avoid It

Alpha-blocker medication (such as Hytrin) and all-natural products such as Prostat have helped many men with BPH, making surgery unnecessary. (See Chapter 7 for more on Prostat.) On the other hand, some men prefer surgery over taking medications for the rest of their lives. Men with more severe symptoms, or those who do not respond to the drugs, may also require surgery.

TRANSURETHRAL INCISION OF THE PROSTATE (TUIP)

Transurethral incision of the prostate (TUIP) is another surgery to relieve symptoms of BPH. TUIP uses the same types of surgical tools as does the "Roto-Rooter" TURP, but instead of removing the offending tissue, the surgeon simply makes one or two long cuts in the prostate tissue. The goal is to "release" the prostatic urethra and neck of the bladder, allowing them to open wider.

A 1990 study reported that TUIP is primarily useful for managing bladder outlet obstruction in "young, middle-aged, and those older men with small prostates who otherwise would be subjected for years to dilatation, massage, and drugs with only partial and temporary relief."[6] The study reports that when TUIP is compared to TURP, the results and complications are the same, except that TURP leads to more contractures of the bladder neck, more reflux ejaculation (sperm going up into the bladder), and increased sexual difficulties.

A 1992 paper reported that "the long-term results of TUIP are quite favorable when compared with those of TURP."[7] TUIP is performed more quickly than is the TURP, and produces little bleeding during the operation and afterward. There's less chance of developing dilutional hyponatremia (also known as the previously mentioned TURP syndrome, caused by absorption of irrigating fluids used during a TURP). TUIP has fewer complications than does the TURP, especially retrograde ejaculation and impotence, and requires less time in the hospital. Since it can be done with local anesthesia, it may be useful for patients whose poor health will not let them withstand the rigors of surgery requiring anesthesia. It's also less expensive than a TURP. Some doctors argue that TUIP will soon replace the TURP as the surgery of choice for relieving bladder obstruction caused by relatively mild degrees of BPH.

Of course, TUIP has its drawbacks. It's not an effective procedure for patients with larger glands (greater than 30 grams in weight), or whose prostates have grown in a particular configuration. And, because no prostatic tissue is removed from the patient and examined in the laboratory, there's no chance to check the tissue for cancer.

We don't yet know enough about the long-term effects of TUIP to say whether or not it will replace the TURP as the "gold standard" surgery for BPH.

TRANSURETHRAL NEEDLE ABLATION OF THE PROSTATE (TUNA)

Transurethral needle ablation of the prostate (TUNA) is a newer attempt to treat BPH with a relatively low cost surgery that's minimally stressful to the patient's body.

TUNA devices use needles incorporated into a special catheter to deliver high-temperature, low-level radio frequency to selected areas of overgrown prostate tissue. The catheter, which is inserted into the penis and pushed up to the prostate, can be guided by direct vision (with the surgeon looking through the catheter) or by ultrasound, with an ultrasound probe inserted into the patient's rectum.

When the device is in place, the needles deliver the radio-frequency heat to small areas of the prostate, destroying the overgrown tissue without damaging the urethra (thanks to adjustable shields on the needles). The needles can be inserted into various portions of the prostate as they "blast out" a widened passageway through which urine can flow unimpeded. Requiring only a local anesthesia, TUNA can be performed as an outpatient procedure.

It's difficult to comment on the efficacy of TUNA because it is so new. If subsequent studies confirm the early enthusiasm for the procedure, TUNA may become a useful, relatively easy and inexpensive surgery for selected BPH patients.

TRANSURETHRAL BALLOON DILATATION (TUBD)

Also known as balloon dilatation of the prostate (BDP) and transurethral dilatation of the prostate (TUDP), TUBD or "the balloon" attempts to treat BPH symptoms by literally pushing them away. A special, uninflated balloon is inserted into the penis under local, regional, or general anesthesia. When the very strong balloon is properly placed in the prostatic urethra, the surgeon inflates it and it squeezes against the overgrown prostate tissue—impeding the flow of urine through the urethra and pushing it out and away (see Figure 5.2). We

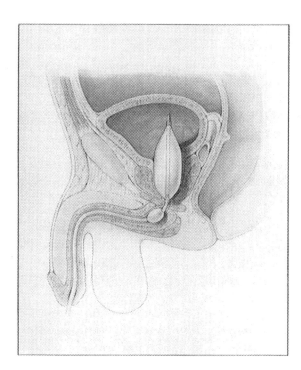

FIGURE 5.2 AMS Optilume™ Prostate Balloon Dilator being inflated in the prostate. *Photo courtesy of American Medical Systems.*

don't know exactly why this works. It may be that (1) compressing the prostate and expelling fluid allows the urethral lumen to enlarge, (2) the muscle tone in the area is changed, or (3) the lobes of the prostate are forcibly separated. It may also be that some other mechanism, or combination of mechanisms, is responsible.

"The balloon" initially generated a great deal of excitement. It seemed, at last, that here was a simple, quick, almost bloodless procedure to relieve BPH symptoms that could be repeated again and again, if necessary, through the years. There would be no incontinence, no impotency, no retrograde ejaculation, and no serious bleeding or infection. Unfortunately, the early promise was not borne out; studies on the balloon have been mixed. Some researchers say it's slightly more effective than a TURP, yet others say it's slightly less effective. In one study, the balloon was compared to catheterization alone, with no balloon at all.[8] (In other words, a catheter was inserted into the patient's penis, but the balloon was not inflated.) The authors of this study concluded that just putting a catheter into the penis was as effective as the catheter with the balloon. They surmised that "the efficacy previously observed after balloon dilatation of the prostate is primarily placebo-related."

Some researchers believe that balloon dilatation of the prostate may be of some value for the temporary relief of mild BPH symptoms in younger men with smaller prostates who wish to postpone having a TURP because they fear the sexual complications. It may also be useful for older men who are suffering from BPH but who are not healthy enough to undergo a TURP. At present, the balloon is not widely used.

LASER-INDUCED PROSTATECTOMY

A great deal of interest has focused on the use of laser beams to reduce BPH symptoms. The idea is to insert a laser probe into the penis and guide it up to the prostatic urethra, where it is fired in order to destroy overgrown tissue obstructing the flow of urine. This causes what is called coagulation necrosis of the prostate. The dead tissue sloughs off and flows out with the urine over the next several weeks.

There are two primary forms of the coagulation necrosis laser-induced prostatectomy: visual laser ablation of the prostate (VLAP) and ultrasound-guided transurethral laser-induced prostatectomy (TULIP).

The surgeon using VLAP, the simpler of the two methods, looks through the combined scope-laser as he pushes it up through the penis to the prostate, then fires the laser at the target tissue. The potential advantages of VLAP are that it is a short procedure, produces less bleeding following the operation, requires minimal time in the hospital, and has fewer side effects. Potential side effects include infection of the urinary tract, swelling of the genitalia, incontinence, impotence, retrograde ejaculation, and strictures of the urethra or bladder neck. Difficulties caused by the laser surgery may later require medications or additional surgery.

The TULIP combines the principles of balloon dilatation and the simple laser. Guided by ultrasound, the surgeon inserts an uninflated balloon through the patient's penis to the prostatic urethra. When the balloon is in place, it's inflated by the surgeon. The prostatic tissue is compressed by the balloon, then fired upon by the laser. The idea between the combined balloon/laser is to squeeze the blood out of the local tissue before firing the laser, thus allowing the laser to penetrate more deeply than it would if the blood had not been squeezed out. The urethral channel widens as dead prostate tissue sloughs off, relieving the patient's urinary difficulties.

Compared to the TURP (the first of the surgeries discussed), TULIP produces very little bleeding, requires less time in the hospital, and is less likely to produce retrograde ejaculation. On the other hand, the TURP removes more tissue than do either of the laser surgeries. TURP produces results almost immediately, whereas a man will have to wait until the tissue sloughs off following a laser surgery. In fact, until the tissue has fallen away, the laser approach may make a man's urinary symptoms temporarily worse.

Because it takes up to six weeks for BPH tissue to slough off and be expelled, patients may not experience any improvement in symptoms for some time after the lasers have been used for "coagulation necrosis." A new approach to laser prostatectomy, using "vaporization," that is currently being developed may eliminate this problem. Instead of allowing dead tissue to remain in place for many weeks, like a rotten apple on a bough, the new approach instantly vaporizes the tissue. Moving the laser back and forth through the prostatic urethra, the surgeon carves out a larger tunnel for the urine to flow through. The results are immediate as the doctor shaves away thin layers of overgrown prostatic tissue—and the tissue simply vaporizes, washing out with the irrigating fluid.

"Vaporization" methods are primitive compared to "coagulation necrosis" techniques, and vaporization surgery takes longer to perform. Although early studies on vaporization are promising, at this point we don't have much data on technique because it is so new.

Dr. Leonard S. Marks of Los Angeles, who so kindly assisted in gathering this information on laser prostatectomy, is currently conducting a pilot study comparing the two approaches—in the same men. Each of the ten to fifteen patients in his study is having one lobe of the prostate treated by "coagulation necrosis," the other with "vaporization." Treating each man with both techniques will allow Dr. Marks to see which approach gives better results, with fewer side effects.

At this point, the various forms of laser prostatectomy show a lot of promise, but are still in the developmental stage.

TWO ALTERNATIVE TREATMENTS

Stents

Researchers have been experimenting with little spiral devices called stents to relieve some of the symptoms of BPH. The first stent was introduced some fifteen years ago as an alternative for men with certain urinary difficulties who were not healthy enough to undergo surgery. Rather than having to have a catheter left in place for long periods of time, they could have a small metal coil placed in the prostatic urethra to hold it open and allow the urine to flow freely.

Often using only local anesthesia, the stent can be placed in less than half an hour. Bleeding is minimal, but the stents can cause urinary urgency, incontinence, and pain. They can also become dislodged. Since we don't yet know what the long-term benefits and drawbacks are, most experts recommend stents only as an alternative to a urethral catheter, or on a temporary basis in patients who are not healthy enough for surgery.

Heat

Heat, also known as hyperthermia or thermotherapy, has been used to treat prostate tissue overgrowth as well as cancerous prostate cells. Researchers report that as many as 80 percent of the men studied had subjective and objective improvement in BPH symptoms following the application of heat. The heat can be applied via either the urethra or the rectum.

Transurethral microwave thermotherapy (TUMT) allows doctors to heat the prostate to high temperatures. A special catheter is threaded through the penis up to the prostatic urethra. An antenna attached to the catheter directs the heat to the appropriate areas of the prostate. The catheter also carries water, which is used to cool the urethra to prevent injury. Proponents of TUMT argue that it is a one-time treatment for patients with moderate or mild BPH and requires no anesthesia. A study[9] of 336 patients with BPH found "significant subjective response" in a majority of the patients, but "[o]bjective improvement was less pronounced." About a quarter of the men developed urinary retention.

Transrectal hyperthermia (THT) delivers heat to the prostate via an antenna built into a special rectal probe. Early results were promising, but it is felt that the higher temperatures possible with the urethral approach make the TUMT superior to the THT for many patients.

As you can see, there are a lot of choices for men to make: Radical prostatectomy, cryosurgery, TURP, TUIP, TUNA, TUDP, VLAP, TULIP, stents, TUMT, THT, and whatever else is currently being developed. Should you need prostate surgery, review each option carefully with your physician before making a decision. And, as previously stated, if your doctor refuses to discuss all the options with you, it's time to start looking for a replacement.

Before discussing other treatments for prostate problems in Chapter 6, let's take a quick look at anesthesia.

A WORD ON ANESTHESIA

Anesthesia is a mysterious and often frightening concept to patients. It's a shame that doctors rarely discuss it with their patients, because a simple conversation can often help to alleviate many fears. It's also a shame that doctors almost never tell their patients that there *may* be a choice of anesthesia, thus allowing patients to participate in a decision-making process that could help them to feel more confident about the surgery.

With perhaps some bias, I asked the best anesthesiologist I know, my son Eric Miller, M.D., of Phoenix, to tell me a little about anesthesia. Here's what he told me:

Before the Surgery . . .

The anesthesiologist should visit or call the patient the day before surgery, for several reasons:

- To review the patient's medical and surgical history.
- To find out if the patient currently has or has had any major systemic diseases such as diabetes, high blood pressure, thyroid disease, heart problems, asthma, or lung disease. The presence of these diseases can affect the way the patient responds to surgery or anesthesia.
- To discuss the patient's prior surgical history: What surgeries he has had, what type of anesthesia was used, and the problems experienced, if any. It's also important to find out if any of the patient's blood relatives have had surgery or anesthesia, and what the results have been. The anesthesiologist is on the lookout for several problems, including a family history of malignant hyperthermia. Malignant hyperthermia is a condition that can cause serious problems during surgery, including severe muscle contraction, significant increases in body temperature, a blood condition called acidosis, kidney failure, dangerous irregular heartbeats, and even death.
- To note the patient's height and weight, and ask if he is allergic to any medications, if he drinks or smokes, and if he uses any illegal drugs. (Although many people are reluctant, it's important that

they admit any use of illegal drugs, because the medicines and gases the anesthesiologist gives before, during, and after surgery can interact with the drugs, causing trouble.)

• To find out which, if any, prescription or over-the-counter medications the patient is taking. The anesthesiologist may ask the patient not to use certain drugs prior to the surgery, or to use less.

Having gathered information, the anesthesiologist should discuss with the patient the type of anesthesia that will be used. Eric explained: "I like to review the type of anesthesia with patients, even though it takes extra time, because it helps to relieve their fears. I find that the more my patients know about what's happening, the better they feel, and the more they cooperate. Another advantage is that the discussion gives me a chance to get to know my patients as people, and for them to see that I really care about them. I want each one to know that he's not just another patient to me—he's a real person, and I'm going to do my best to help him sail through the surgery."

Two types of anesthesia are used for most prostate surgeries: general and what we call "regional." With general anesthesia, patients are put into a comatose state. With regional anesthesia, only regions (parts) of the body are anesthetized.

Surgery with General Anesthesia

The morning of the surgery, the anesthesiologist should meet the patient in the preoperative area. An IV (intravenous) line is started by the anesthesiologist or a nurse. The patient is usually given a sedative (what Eric calls a "Margarita") to make him comfortable.

Then the patient is taken into the operating suite, and transferred from the gurney to the operating table. The operating suite is usually chilly, so the patient is covered with warm blankets (which have been preheated and feel as if they're warm from the dryer). The anesthesiologist attaches heart, blood pressure, and blood oxygen monitors to the patient. Depending on the type of surgery, and on the patient's physical and health status, other monitors may be required. "The monitors let us see into the patient's body to let us know what's happening," Eric says. "It is critical that we have this constantly updated information."

When the patient has been fully prepared, the induction period begins. The patient is given more medication to sedate him, and 100 percent oxygen to breathe from a face mask. Then he's given drugs to put him completely out; he enters a comatose state. This is a crucial period, for the drugs have depressed the patient's respiratory drive to the point at which he can't breathe on his own. Working quickly, the anesthesiologist must place an endotrachial tube into the patient's mouth, past the vocal cords, and into the trachea. With the tube in place, the patient's breathing is controlled by a mechanical ventilator. With the patient's breathing safely handled by machine, the anesthesiologist can give additional medicines to make sure that the patient stays properly anesthetized.

During the surgery, the anesthesiologist watches the patient and the various monitors carefully, making sure that things such as breathing, pulse, oxygen saturation of the blood, body temperature, and body position are proper. The patient's body position is very important because improper positioning can cause nerve damage as well as other problems.

As the surgery comes to a close, the anesthesiologist begins to taper off, or turn off, the anesthesia. "Waking patients up at the proper time is the real art of anesthesia," says Eric. "You want the patient to be semi-awake and breathing on his own by the time the surgeon has closed the incision and is putting on the dressing."

When the patient is breathing well on his own and is awake enough, he's transferred to a gurney and wheeled into the postanesthesia care unit (what used to be called the recovery room). There, the anesthesiologist hands the patient over to nurses, who hook the patient up to monitoring devices. The anesthesiologist writes up a report, informing the nurses of potential complications, and tells them what medications—such as those for pain and nausea—are being prescribed for the patient.

Surgery with "Regional" Anesthesia

Regional anesthesia is designed to affect only specific regions of the body—for example, the area from the waist down. We may use regional anesthesia for transurethral resection of the prostate (TURP) or other "smaller" surgeries. There are two regional procedures used for prostate surgeries: spinal anesthesia and epidural anesthesia.

Spinal anesthesia is injected directly into the patient's spinal canal. First the anesthesiologist scrubs the patient's back with a soapy solution, then injects a local anesthesia. When the area is numb, the anesthesiologist pushes a needle into the patient's spinal canal, between the bones of the back. When the needle is in the spinal canal, spinal fluid will be observed dripping out of the needle. When the needle is in place, the anesthesiologist attaches a syringe full of the medication and injects the drug, which should begin taking effect within seconds. During surgery, the anesthesiologist monitors the patient very carefully. Following surgery, the anesthesia is allowed to wear off naturally.

With epidural anesthesia, a larger needle is used to inject drugs into the epidural space around the spinal canal. The medicine then diffuses (spreads) into the spinal canal. An epidural requires more medicine and is slower to take effect, but is easier to control. The epidural needle is carefully manipulated by the anesthesiologist, who uses touch and the feeling of resistance to guide the needle into place. By continuously applying controlled pressure to the plunger, the anesthesiologist can tell when the needle is in the epidural space because the plunger is then easy to depress. To make sure the needle is in the epidural space, and not in the spinal canal, the anesthesiologist injects a test dose of medicine. If the epidural takes effect immediately, there is a cessation of pain. The doctor verifies by testing the patient's pain response. Also, if he sees any spinal fluid, he knows he's in the wrong area. If everything looks OK, the anesthesiologist pushes down on the plunger and gives the patient the full dose. During surgery, the anesthesiologist monitors the patient very carefully. Following surgery, the anesthesia is allowed to wear off naturally.

With either spinal or epidural anesthesia, the effects of the anesthesia may go all the way up to the patient's belly button. His legs feel very heavy. He might be able to feel pressure, but not pain, in his legs. The patient may also be given a slight sedative for relaxation. He will still be able to respond to commands, and can usually complain of major pain—which may signal a surgical error. The patient is also usually given oxygen through a mask or nasal prongs.

The spinal is easier to do, and takes effect sooner. The epidural may be used for longer surgeries. A catheter may be placed into the epidural space, allowing the anesthesiologist to give more anesthesia during the surgery, as well as pain medications afterward.

Now that you know what to expect from your surgery and anesthesia, Chapter 6 presents some other treatments for prostate problems, including radiation and hormone therapy.

6

Other Standard Treatments for Prostate Problems

Many men wish to avoid surgery, and for good reason. Despite the benefits of prostate surgery, it is not always the best solution. And even when surgery is indicated, some men are, understandably, too frightened to agree to the procedure. Fortunately, other therapies are available. We'll look first at the two main categories of treatment for prostate cancer—hormonal and radiation therapy—then examine an emerging approach called hyperthermia. The chapter will conclude with a brief look at chemotherapy, and a discussion of what is called "watchful waiting."

HORMONE THERAPY

The cancer cells growing in the prostate are hungry, and one of the "foods" they need in order to grow is testosterone, the male sex hormone. Taking the point even further, some call testosterone the "fertilizer" for prostate cancer. Hormone therapy attacks prostate cancer by taking away its "fertilizer." In fact, Drs. Huggins and Hodges won the Nobel Prize in 1953 for their discovery that eliminating testosterone caused regression of prostate cancer.

Since most of the testosterone in a man's body is made by his testicles, an early approach consisted of removing the testicles in order to starve the cancer of testosterone. The surgical removal of one testicle is called an orchiectomy; removal of both is a bilateral (both sides) orchiectomy. Even though this is a surgery, it is considered a hormone therapy since the hormone output is drastically reduced. This very logical approach—removing the testicles and stopping the adrenal

102

testosterone—is obviously unacceptable to many men. Or, if they do accept the treatment, they may suffer severe psychological side effects.

But there's another source of testosterone in the body. The two adrenal glands, one sitting atop each kidney, also produce small amounts of testosterone (5 to 10 percent of a man's total output). Removing the testicles is not enough: The testosterone coming from the adrenal glands must also be stopped.

Fortunately, there are ways of cutting off the flow of testosterone from the testicles and adrenal glands without surgically removing them. Certain substances can block the flow or the conversion of testosterone. In addition to orchiectomy, techniques of hormone therapy are:

- LHRH agents that block the testicular testosterone. The use of these medicines is sometimes referred to as a "medical orchiectomy."
- Antiandrogens to block the adrenal testosterone.
- Estrogen to block testosterone.

Hormone Therapy #1: Orchiectomy

Doctors describe the orchiectomy as a "minor procedure," but most patients would not describe it as such. The surgery is performed through an incision in the scrotum. The entire testis may be removed, or, in a procedure called a subcapsular orchiectomy, it may be cored out and the outer shell left in place. A prosthetic device similar to silicon breast implants can be implanted to make it appear as if the man's testes are still there. *The orchiectomy only removes the testes. The scrotum (the skin pouch holding the testes) and the penis are left intact.*

The orchiectomy removes the major source of testosterone, striking an important blow against the prostate cancer. It's a one-time procedure; you don't have to keep going back to the doctor's office for more treatment, and you won't have to take shots. Once it's done, it's done.

Given a choice, however, many men would prefer to keep their testicles, opting instead for a treatment that will stop the testicular testosterone without surgery. LHRH injections do just that.

Hormone Therapy #2: Medical Orchiectomy

LHRH (luteinizing hormone-releasing hormone) agonists are medications that turn off the flow of testosterone from the testicles. The treatment, which consists of monthly injections, is often called a "medical orchiectomy" or "medical castration" because the medicine mimics the effects of the surgery.

How do the hormones work? The process begins in the pituitary gland, a part of the brain. The pituitary uses LHRH to stimulate the Leydig cells, cells inside the testes that secrete testosterone. LHRH agonists (enemies) interfere with the LHRH, making it impossible for the pituitary to signal the testes to produce testosterone. The testicles are still in place, but they're not getting the "order" to make testosterone.

The advantage of LHRH agonist therapy is obvious to men: You get to keep your testicles. The disadvantages have to do with convenience and cost. You must go back to your doctor's office once a month for your injection, and the injections cost a lot of money. (Researchers are trying to develop longer-lasting injections.) However, unlike the orchiectomy, LHRH agonist therapy is reversible: You can drop the therapy and try another form of treatment.

Lupron and Zoladex are two of the LHRH agonists.

Lupron injection

Chemical name: Leuprolide acetate

How administered: As an injection

Uses: For the palliative treatment of advanced cancer of the prostate. Leupron reduces symptoms but does not cure the cancer.

When you take Lupron: Your testosterone levels will go up at first, possibly worsening your symptoms. Within two weeks, however, your testosterone levels should be back to where they were when you began taking the drug, and should continue to drop.

Adverse reactions: Rising testosterone levels in the majority of patients during the first week or so may increase symptoms, including bone pain (if present). There have been a few reported cases of blood in the urine (hematuria) and obstruction of the urinary tract during the first week, as well as temporary weakness and other problems.

Other possible adverse reactions include angina, cardiac arrhythmias, myocardial infarction, pulmonary emboli, diarrhea, gastrointestinal bleeding, peptic ulcer, rectal polyps, decrease in libido, enlargement of the thyroid, joint pain, anxiety, blurred vision, lethargy, mood swings, nervousness, numbness, peripheral neuropathy, blackouts, cough, pneumonia, pulmonary fibrosis, carcinoma of the skin/ear, dry skin, hair loss, bladder spasms, incontinence, pain in the testicles, depression, diabetes, fatigue, fever, and blood changes.

A number of patients on Lupron have developed marked fatigue, senile features, and depression, all of which improved after they stopped taking the medication. There are also the adverse effects caused by the drop in testosterone, including shrinking of the testicles, hot flashes, and impotence.

Recommended dose: Lupron Depot (long-acting), 7.5 mg, is given by injection into muscle once a month.

Zoladex

Chemical name: Goserelin acetate implant

How administered: As an injection

Uses: The palliative treatment of advanced cancer of the prostate. Zoladex reduces symptoms but does not cure the cancer.

When you take Zoladex: Your testosterone levels will go up at first, possibly worsening your symptoms for the first few weeks only.

Adverse reactions: Rising testosterone levels in the majority of patients during the early stages of treatment may increase symptoms, including bone pain (if present). Other possible adverse reactions include cardiac arrhythmias, stroke, hypertension, myocardial infarction, chest pain, anxiety, depression, headaches, constipation, diarrhea, ulcers, vomiting, anemia, gout, weight increase, chills, fever, urinary tract infection, breast tenderness, and swelling.

There are also the adverse effects caused by the drop in testosterone, including the shrinking of the testicles, hot flashes, and impotence.

Recommended dose: The recommended dose for Zoladex is 3.6 mg, injected every 28 days. The dose is administered subcutaneously (under the skin) into the abdominal wall.

Zoladex versus orchiectomy: Zoladex has been compared to orchiectomy in a controlled study for patients with advanced prostate cancer. The long-term objective responses and length of survival were similar.[1]

Hormone Therapy #3:
Antiandrogens for the Adrenals

Orchiectomy or LHRH injections handle the testosterone coming from the testicles, but something is still needed to handle the much smaller amounts of testosterone coming from the adrenal glands.

The medicines that attack this part of the problem are called antiandrogens. (Androgens are substances that increase male characteristics.) Because the adrenal glands produce such a small proportion of the total testosterone, antiandrogen therapy by itself is not effective. It must be done as part of a complete testosterone blockage therapy. Using LHRH agonists to block testicular testosterone, together with antiandrogens to stop adrenal testosterone, is called "complete androgen blockage" or "combined androgen deprivation."

The antiandrogens (taken in pill and tablet form) are very effective, but the pills must be taken several times a day and are quite expensive. However, unlike the orchiectomy, antiandrogen therapy is reversible. You can drop the therapy in favor of another if you desire.

Eulexin, Cytadren, and Nizoral are antiandrogens.

Eulexin

Chemical name: Flutamide

How administered: Orally, as capsules. It is used in conjunction with an LHRH agonist to treat cancer that has spread beyond the prostate.

Adverse reactions: Flutamide and LHRH agonists given together produced hot flashes, loss of libido, impotence, diarrhea, nausea and vomiting, gynecomastia, and gastrointestinal disturbances. When given with LHRH agonists, flutamide may cause hypertension, drowsiness, anxiety, confusion, anorexia, anemia, and other problems.

Recommended dose: The recommended dose for Eulexin capsules is 750 mg a day. Patients take two capsules three times a day at eight-hour intervals.

Cytadren

Chemical name: Aminoglutethimide

Note: Cytadren is generally used to suppress adrenal function in certain patients with Cushing's syndrome.

How administered: Orally, as tablets

Adverse reactions: Cytadren works strongly against adrenal hormones. It is so powerful, in fact, that men taking the drug must also be given cortisone to prevent adrenal insufficiency. Other possible adverse effects seen in patients treated for Cushing's syndrome include drowsiness, skin rash, nausea, anorexia, dizziness, blood changes, headaches, hypotension, vomiting, abnormal liver function tests, fever, delayed healing, and a tendency toward bruising.

Nizoral

Chemical name: Ketoconazole

Note: Nizoral cream was originally used to fight fungus. When it was discovered that Nizoral also inhibited adrenal hormones, it was used in patients whose cancer had spread to the spine, or when orchiectomy had not worked.

Hormone Therapy #4: Estrogens

Taking estrogen, the female hormone, also stops the production of testicular testosterone. Diethylstilbestrol, also known as DES, is a synthetic estrogen used for prostate cancer that has either spread or returned.

Estrogen therapy was largely abandoned in the United States because it increased the risk of heart disease. The estrogen dosages have been refined and reduced in recent years, however, thereby lowering that accompanying risk. As estrogens become safer, and as costs become more important to the U.S. medical system, this relatively inexpensive hormone therapy may make a comeback in the treatment of prostate cancer.

Estrogens are indicated for cancer that is progressing but is inoperable. Possible adverse reactions include nausea, vomiting, headaches, pain in the abdomen, enlargement of the breasts, bloating, loss of appetite, skin rash, depression, nervousness, dizziness, pain in the chest, shortness of breath, frequent urination, and pain upon urination. Thrombophlebitis, pulmonary embolisms, cerebral thrombosis, and impotence have also been associated with the use of estrogens.

Comparing Hormone Therapies

Treatment	What It Does	Pros	Cons
Orchiectomy	Surgically eliminates the major source of testosterone.	A relatively simple, inexpensive surgery. Permanent.	All surgeries are risky. Irreversible. There are physical side effects, and the psychological effects may be severe.
LHRH Therapy	Significantly decreases production of testosterone.	No surgery involved, only injections. Reversible.	Expensive monthly shots required. Has various physical and psychological side effects, including possibly a temporary increase of symptoms.
Antiandrogen Therapy	Blocks testosterone activity.	No surgery involved, only pills. Reversible.	Various physical and psychological side effects. Patient must continue on pills for as long as therapy continues.
Estrogen Therapy	Decreases production of testosterone.	No surgery involved, only pills. Reversible. Relatively inexpensive.	Various physical and psychological side effects.

Who Should Have Hormone Therapy?

When orchiectomy was the only form of hormone therapy available, it was reserved for only advanced cases. With the advent of new medications, however, hormone therapy is being used in earlier stages.

If the cancer is confined to the prostate, and the doctors feel it can be successfully and totally removed surgically, hormone therapy is not indicated—unless the patient's health precludes surgery. Some doctors also use hormone therapy before surgery or radiation, in an attempt to shrink the tumor and make the procedures more successful. We don't really know if this is truly helpful or not.

There is a great deal of controversy concerning what to do if the cancer has spread from the prostate to local or distant tissues. Surgery, radiation, hormone treatment, and combinations of the three are all recommended by various authorities. Recommendations for you will depend upon your age, general health, and your doctor's particular preferences. Whatever is recommended, make sure that you are advised of all the possible treatments, and that *your* preferences are carefully considered as well.

The Psychophysiological Side Effects of Hormone Therapy

While not life-threatening, the side effects of hormone therapy are disturbing to many men. Interfering with testosterone, the male sex hormone, reduces a man's desire for sexual relations, as well as his ability to get or keep an erection; a loss of muscle mass and fatigue are common; many men also experience hot flashes, and some suffer gastrointestinal symptoms. There are medicines to deal with the hot flashes and gastrointestinal symptoms, and there are treatments for impotence. Whereas some men are able to continue enjoying sexual intercourse during hormonal therapy, others are psychologically devastated by the "loss of their manhood."

The End Result of Hormone Therapy

While hormone therapy can effectively halt the spread of cancer for some time, and even cause shrinkage of the tumor, prostate cancer cells eventually "learn" how to continue growing with only very little amounts of testosterone, or, apparently, without any at all. It may be that the cancer cells eventually become immune to the therapy. Or perhaps the hormone therapy kills the bulk of the cancer cells, but those few that don't need testosterone multiply to the point at which they become dangerous once again. When that happens, hormone therapy is no longer effective.

RADIATION THERAPY

When I was a child, the shoe salesman had an interesting way to prove to my mother that his shoes fit me perfectly. He would literally X-ray my feet while I was wearing his shoes. We kids had a ball with that machine, playfully visualizing the bones of our feet, never realizing that we were exposing ourselves to cancer-causing X rays.

Radiation therapy, also called radiotherapy or irradiation, attempts to treat cancer by irradiating the cancerous cells to death, thus preventing them from growing and dividing. The idea is to kill off enough of the cancerous growth to shrink it, thereby making it less dangerous, reducing any pressure it might be placing on other parts of the body, and possibly reducing pain, bleeding, or other symptoms. *However, be aware that radiation therapy does not cure cancer that has spread beyond the prostate.*

Two approaches are used to deliver the radiation: External beam and internal seeds.

Radiation Therapy #1: External Beam Radiation

External beam radiation is what most people think of when they hear the word "radiation." We picture someone lying on a cold, hard table surrounded by tons of intimidating machinery. A technician pulls a huge arm of the machine over his body, and adjusts a few dials. The machinery hums for a little while, then it's all over.

The classic work on the use of external radiation to treat prostate cancer was done by Dr. Bagshaw at Stanford. Radiologists feel that radiation is at least as good as surgery for treating prostate cancer, with fewer side effects. (Surgeons, of course, dispute these findings. They think that surgery is the best approach.)

Radiation works by killing cells when they attempt to divide. If you take a biopsy of the prostate right after radiation, you'll see cancer cells that seem to be intact. However, they can't divide and multiply, so they eventually die off. This explains why some tumors may shrink slowly with radiation—it takes a while for all of the cells to get to the point of dividing. Because of this, the tumor will continue shrinking, and the PSA should continue falling, after the radiation therapy is completed. (The PSA may actually rise when the therapy begins, due to cellular destruction.)

Radiation therapy typically begins by treating an area wider than the projected size of the cancer. The idea is that it's better to radiate a little too much, and make sure that all the cancer is gone, rather than risk the regrowth of the cancer by letting even a few cells escape. The machine that delivers the radiation can be adjusted to "hit" the patient from various angles, including from below. Protective shields will be placed over other parts of the body for protection from the radiation. Generally speaking, the smaller the cancer, the easier the cure.

Handling the Side Effects of Radiation

For Fatigue—Get as much rest as possible. You may have to take time off from work, or work part-time during your treatment. To help keep your strength up, eat as healthful a diet as possible. (See Chapter 11 for more on diet.)

For Nausea—In addition to medications to combat nausea, you can try either not eating anything right before your treatment, or eating just a small amount of bland food such as crackers or toast; eating small meals; drinking cool liquids between meals; or eating easy-to-digest foods such as clear broth and dry toast. If you begin to feel nauseated, try breathing slowly and deeply, and distracting yourself with television, conversation, or music. Relaxation techniques are helpful.

For Diarrhea—In addition to taking medicines for diarrhea, you can try avoiding coffee, tea, alcohol, sweets, fried foods, and greasy and highly spiced foods; eating frequent small meals; switching to lower-fiber foods such as white bread and rice, mashed potatoes, skinless turkey or chicken, or canned or cooked fruit without the skin. Be sure to drink plenty of liquids to replace the fluid you lose due to diarrhea. Unless otherwise instructed, eat good amounts of bananas, oranges, potatoes, peaches, and other potassium-rich foods to help replace the potassium lost in your stool. Avoid milk and milk products if you are allergic or sensitive to them; they can worsen diarrhea in sensitive people.

For Skin Irritation—Wear loose clothing over the radiated area, don't rub or scratch the area; don't use soaps, lotions, powders, perfumes, or other potions on the area; stop using starch or any laundry soaps or other preparations that may irritate you; ask your doctor to recommend any special lotions or medicines that might be helpful. You may want to try aloe vera lotions or creams, which have been used for radiation burns since the 1930s.

(For information on urinary and sexual difficulties, see Chapter 9.)

If the cancer has spread beyond the local area, radiation cannot offer a cure. It is often used to help relieve symptoms, including the pain caused by cancer that has spread to the bones. Relatively small doses of radiation directed to small, specific areas can shrink a tumor that is causing pain. However, there are usually too many of these "small" cancers spread throughout the body, and unfortunately, radiation can't kill them all.

For localized prostate cancer, the course of treatment usually runs six to eight weeks, five days a week. There are several schools of thought concerning the duration of the treatment, as well as how tightly the radiation should be focused upon the cancer. Some doctors treat wider areas, some narrower.

Should the radiation fail to eradicate the cancer, alternatives are surgery, cryosurgery, hyperthermia, and hormones. However, you cannot have a repeat course of radiation, since too much radiation can actually cause cancer.

Some men can't tolerate radiation at all if their general health is poor, they've had prior surgery in the area, their intestines are too near the radiation field, or other reasons. And some people are simply too sensitive to radiation to withstand the treatment.

Drawbacks

One of the main drawbacks of radiation therapy is that we can't be absolutely certain that the cancer has been completely eliminated. The therapy will often push PSA levels way down, but in a disturbing number of cases the PSA begins to rise again several years later. Another drawback to radiation therapy is the very real possibility that the nerve adjacent to the prostate may be damaged, leading to impotence.

Side effects of external beam radiation therapy include fatigue, nausea, diarrhea, skin irritation and radiation skin burns, and urinary and sexual difficulties.

Radiation Therapy #2:
Internal Seed Radiation

A new method developed in the early 1970s was called internal radiation, or radiation implants. Instead of hitting the patient with a radioactive beam, the doctors actually implanted little radioactive "seeds" inside the prostate. The idea was to get small doses of the radiation exactly where it was needed, without having to pass through other parts of the body, and without the risk of "overshooting" or missing the target. Cancerous cells near the implant die and are eliminated by the body.

The early work with radiation implants was not terribly successful, partially because doctors had to literally open the patient up in order to implant the radioactive seeds into the prostate. Then they had to "feel their way around" the prostate and guess as to the best spots for implanting the seeds. Some patients wound up with too many seeds and too much radiation in some areas of the prostate, but not enough seeds or radiation in other areas.

Today, the seeds are implanted through small needles pushed into the prostate via the perineum (the area between the scrotum and the rectum). Guided by images created by an ultrasound probe placed in the patient's rectum, the doctor inserts perhaps fifty to eighty seeds. The modern procedure is less traumatic than the older surgical implant, and the seeds are more accurately placed.

The actual seeds are like little pieces of rice or birdseed. (See Figure 6.1 to get an idea of how small the seeds are.) You can lay many of them on a dime, with room to spare. Some seeds give a relatively short, powerful dose of radiation. Others last longer, while delivering a lower dose.

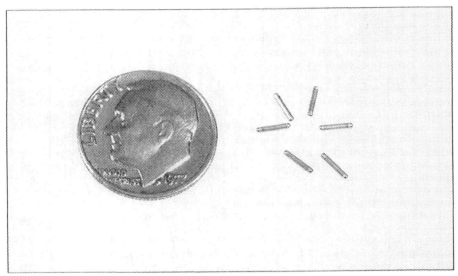

FIGURE 6.1 Iodine-125 seeds next to a dime. Radioactive seeds are implanted into the prostate to kill cancer cells. *Photo courtesy of Amersham Healthcare.*

Good candidates for internal radiation seeds are men with early-stage or small cancers confined to one lobe of the prostate, with PSAs of less than 20, and Gleason scores of 7 or less.[2] The prostate itself should not be much larger than 70 grams or so.

The advantages of radiation seeds are:

- It is an outpatient procedure that takes an hour or two to perform. Skilled doctors can take a pelvic lymph-node biopsy, study the results, and then implant the seeds in two to three hours.
- Recovery can be relatively quick, with patients back at work and engaging in usual activities within several days. (Patients are generally instructed to avoid strenuous physical activity and heavy lifting for a few days after the implantation.)
- The seeds are placed close to or at the cancer site, where they can deliver a concentrated dose of radiation.
- Early studies suggest that rates of incontinence and impotence may be lower with the seeds than with other means.

Before a typical seed implantation, the man will undergo transrectal ultrasound in order to evaluate his prostate. That information is used to prepare a treatment plan—how many seeds are needed, the dosage, and so forth.

The morning of the procedure, the patient will check into the hospital and be taken to the surgical suite. He may be placed under general or spinal anesthesia, depending upon his and the anesthesiologist's preferences. Since the needles will be inserted through the man's perineum, he is placed on his back on the table, with his legs elevated in stirrups. The perineum is prepped and shaved.

A small grid is put in place, an inch or so away from the man's perineum. Made of metal or plastic, the grid has many little holes in it, like Peg-Board. The first needle is placed into the proper hole in the grid. Guided by the ultrasound screen, the doctor carefully pushes the needle through the skin and into the prostate. One by one, the doctor puts all the needles into place, watching carefully to make sure that no needle gets too close to the bladder or rectum.

The number of needles used, usually between ten and twenty, depends upon the size of the patient's prostate. There may be some bleeding from the puncture wounds, but in most cases the patient loses less than 5 cc of blood during the whole procedure.

After the Seed Implantation

This information is taken from the Patient Discharge Instruction sheet given by Arnold Malcolm, M.D., of the St. Joseph Medical Center in Burbank, California, to his patients who have just had seeds implanted in their prostates. *(This information is presented for educational purposes only. It is not to be construed as instructions for your implantation. Please consult your physician for your instructions should you undergo seed implantation.)*

Diet: Regular diet, unless you are on a special diet for other medical reasons.

Activities: Avoid heavy lifting or strenuous physical activity for one week once you have returned home. Thereafter, you may return to your normal physical activity.

Possible Side Effects: Immediately after the surgery, you may experience slight bleeding beneath the scrotum, blood in the urine, and bruising and tenderness between the legs. These side effects are not unusual. They are the result of the implantation of needles into the perineum. Slight discomfort is not unusual; however, if there is excessive bleeding, with blood clots or severe pain, call your physician. Intake of plenty of fluids helps to flush the bladder, and decreases the chances of blood clots forming within the bladder. Burning after the catheter is removed is not unusual. If it persists longer than 6 to 8 hours after the catheter has been removed, contact your urologist.

Possible later side effects include frequent urination, burning with urination, a sense of urinary urgency, and a weaker urinary stream. The surgical procedure and radioactive seeds may cause local swelling of the prostatic tissue, resulting in the above-noted symptoms. Drinking plenty of water helps to relieve these symptoms. Avoiding beverages containing caffeine also helps. If the symptoms are significant, contact your urologist.

(continued)

(Continued from previous page)

Radiation Precautions: Radiation is a concern for many of our patients. The radioactive isotopes used, iodine-125 or palladium-103, are low-energy radioactive sources. This means that, for the most part, the radiation is contained within the prostatic gland. Some radiation reaches adjacent organs, such as the bladder and the rectum. The precautions below are to ensure that those around you are protected from unnecessary radiation.

- *Objects that you touch or wear are not radioactive.*
- *Your bodily waste (urine and stool) is not radioactive.*
- Any pregnant women, or women who might be pregnant, should avoid prolonged, close contact with you for the first two months following the implantation. They should remain at least six feet away from you. There is no limit to the amount of time they may spend in the same room with you.
- Children should not sit on your lap for the first two months following the implant.
- Sexual intercourse may be resumed two weeks following the implant. A condom should be used. Use of a condom can be discontinued two months after the implant.
- Sperm or ejaculate may be discolored (black or brown).
- For about two weeks after removal of the urinary catheter, you may find a few loose seeds in your ejaculate or urine. Recover the seed using forceps or tweezers, place it in aluminum foil, and wrap it up. Return the seed(s) to the physics department of the hospital's radiation oncology unit.

When the needles are all in position, the seeds are placed into the needles. There may be several seeds in one needle, again depending upon the size and shape of the man's prostate. The seeds are then implanted and the needles are pulled back. Stitches are usually not required to close the small puncture wounds.

With the seeds in place, the doctor double-checks everything with the ultrasound. Then a urologist uses a cystoscope to make sure that no seeds have been accidentally placed inside the bladder. (If so, they must be removed.)

The man is then taken to a recovery room. When he's fully awake and feeling fine, the catheter has been removed, and he can urinate on his own, he is free to go home. Most men are able to leave the hospital within four to eight hours of the implantation.

The radioactive seeds in the prostate kill the cancer cells, which the body will then eliminate.

As with all radiation therapies, internal radiation carries with it certain disadvantages. Potential side effects include frequent urination, burning upon urination, uncomfortable urination, blood in the urine, swelling of the testicles, and bleeding or burning in the area beneath the scrotum. Rectal irritation and bleeding have also been seen, as well as discomfort when moving the bowels. Although the rates of incontinence and impotence *may* be somewhat lower than with other radiation therapies, the procedure is too new for us to tell whether it will affect a man's long-term chances of survival. Preliminary results look good: Only time will tell if internal radiation is more accurate, more powerful, and/or less harmful to the patient than is external beam radiation.

Special Caution: It is possible for small amounts of radiation from the seeds to "leak" out of your body. Although most doctors will tell you that it's nothing to worry about, I would suggest that precautions be taken when around pregnant women and small children. (See radiation precautions on pages 115–16.)

HYPERTHERMIA

In Chapter 5, we discussed cryosurgery (freezing) as a possible treatment for prostate problems. We also included hyperthermia[3] (heat) as an alternative approach being used. Although approved in the United States only in the 1980s, hyperthermia has generated a great deal of interest—and controversy.

Hyper- means "over" or "excessive," and *thermia* refers to heat. It's an old idea: Ancient Egyptian physicians used heat to treat patients with smallpox, tuberculosis, gallstones, and breast cancer, among other problems. In the fifth century B.C., Hippocrates, the father of Western medicine, suggested using heat on small tumors.

Hyperthermia by itself is not terribly effective in fighting prostate cancer, but if it is combined with a small dose of radiation, the response can be very good. Some doctors advocate heat plus smaller-than-usual doses of radiation, while others argue that heat plus normal doses of radiation is the most beneficial approach.

Hyperthermia is more widely studied and used in Europe, Japan, and Israel than it is in the United States.

How Hyperthermia Works

No one knows exactly how hyperthermia, in combination with radiation, shrinks tumors. Several theories have been advanced, including:

1. *The Blood Vessel Theory*—All cells, including cancerous ones, need generous supplies of blood in order to remain alive. Due to some unknown weakness, the blood vessels in tumorous areas are more susceptible to heat than are normal vessels. When heat is applied, the blood vessels in the cancerous areas are damaged, and the cancer cells die from lack of blood flow.

2. *The Cellular Damage Theory*—Radiation itself does not kill all of the cancerous cells. Some are only damaged, and can use certain cellular enzymes to repair themselves. These enzymes, however, are sensitive to heat. Hyperthermia stops the repair process by disrupting the enzymes, thus making the radiation treatment more effective.

3. *The Combination Theory*—Radiation and hyperthermia strengthen each other by working on different phases of the cell replication cycle. Radiation works against cells when they are dividing, while hyperthermia works on cells that are stationary. The combination of heat and radiation gives you two ways to attack the cancer cells, instead of only one.

Still other theories of how heat kills or weakens the cancerous cells include: (1) It damages the cells' ability to "breathe," (2) it liberates little "poison packets" (lysozymes) within the cells, (3) it alters the cells' ability to manufacture protein, and (4) it makes the cell walls more permeable, allowing the wrong substances to move in or out of the cells.

How It's Done

The full hyperthermia treatment begins with radiation therapy, which is applied in the same way as external beam radiation. The patient lies on his back on a table, surrounded by rather imposing-looking machinery. The radiation beam is aimed into one or more carefully selected areas in or around the prostate. Depending upon the location, size, and stage of the cancer, the beam may be narrowly focused on the prostate, or it may be widened in an attempt to kill cancer cells that have spread locally.

After radiation, the patient is taken to another room for the hyperthermia treatment. Again, the patient lies on his back. A heating element that looks a little bit like a cigar box is placed between his legs or on his abdomen. A temperature probe, smaller than a pipe cleaner, may be inserted into his rectum to help the doctor monitor the amount of heat that is being applied. Temperature probes may also be attached to the skin. The patient may nap or read during the treatment, which lasts up to an hour. (Figure 6.2 shows what a typical hyperthermia apparatus looks like.)

Either ultrasound or microwaves are used to apply heat at between 107° and 113° Fahrenheit. If ultrasound is used, the technician will apply a gel-like substance to the body, and then place the applicator against the gel (as is done during ultrasounds on pregnant women).

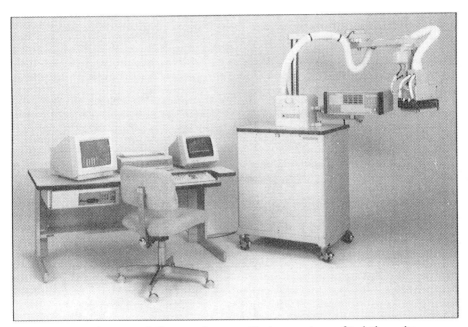

FIGURE 6.2 Ultrasound Therapy System. *Photo courtesy of Labthermics Technologies, Inc.*

A patient typically feels warm all over as his body temperature rises a degree or two. He may also feel warmth between his legs or on his abdomen, depending upon where the heating element has been applied.

Patients typically spend a couple of hours at the doctor's office when receiving the radiation and heat treatments. They will receive the heat and radiation five days a week for six to eight weeks. Except for the temperature probe, the treatment is noninvasive (meaning that the patient's body is not entered). Patients may go home immediately after treatment and continue with their normal activities, unless they feel weak or otherwise ill. They are advised to drink plenty of fluids; some doctors also prescribe Gatorade or a similar drink.

Benefits of Hyperthermia

Numbers are difficult to pin down, but it appears that the combined heat/radiation treatment is an effective tool in the war on prostate cancer. Since the combined heat/radiation treatment uses smaller doses of radiation than does radiation alone, patients generally have fewer radiation-induced side effects. Unlike radiation, which itself is capable of *causing* cancer, hyperthermia does not appear to induce cancer.[4] Hyperthermia has also been used for patients whose cancers have resisted radiation therapy.

Although we used to feel that once a patient's prostate had been radiated it could not be operated upon, some doctors are now arguing that patients can move on to surgery (as well as cryosurgery or hormone therapy) should their hyperthermia fail. This is due to the lower levels of radiation received with hyperthermia. Patients cannot, however, try stand-alone radiation after hyperthermia, because they've already been exposed to a great deal of radiation.

Drawbacks of Hyperthermia

As previously indicated, patients typically feel warmth in the affected area (between the legs or on the abdomen) during hyperthermia treatment. They may feel warm all over, and may sweat, as body temperature rises a degree or two. Toward the end of the treatment series, they may have soreness or a rash between the legs or on the abdomen. They may also develop diarrhea. Another drawback is the fact that patients must go to the doctor's office for treatment five days a week, for six to eight weeks.

Hyperthermia is best used when the cancer is confined to the prostate, or has only spread very locally. Once the cancer has spread to distant areas, hyperthermia cannot cure the patient. Some people have an allergylike reaction to radiation, and cannot have hyperthermia.

Hyperthermia for BPH and Prostatitis

Doctors in Europe, Japan, and Israel have used hyperthermia alone (without radiation) in the treatment of BPH. The heat reduces the gland by up to 20 percent. Studies have been conducted looking at the use of heat in the treatment of prostatitis, but it is too early to tell if this will emerge as a major treatment.

CHEMOTHERAPY

Chemotherapy is a chemical attack on cancer cells. It employs powerful drugs that circulate throughout the entire body, looking for rapidly growing cells, such as cancer cells, to kill. Unfortunately, cancer cells aren't the only ones that grow rapidly: Hair cells, cells lining the stomach, bone marrow cells, and immune-system cells are also rapid growers, and thus are at risk.

Unfortunately, chemotherapy works in only a limited way for men with prostate cancer. At best, it helps relieve some of the symptoms of advanced cancer, but it is not a cure. Side effects include nausea, vomiting, hair loss, an increased risk of infection, and changes to the blood.

ANOTHER APPROACH: "WATCHFUL WAITING"

When I was a student, the older doctors introduced me to the "watchful waiting" approach, also known as "expectant management." The philosophy underlying this approach can be boiled down to one question: Is doing something truly better than simply keeping a careful watch on the situation?

"Watchful waiting"—monitoring but not treating the cancer—is the simplest, least dangerous approach. I say that it is the least dangerous because in only about 3 percent of all cases will prostate cancer invade the surrounding tissues and bone, becoming deadly. *If this happens, however, the results are disastrous.* On the other hand, we know that the overwhelming majority of men die *with* prostate cancer rather than *of* it. We also know that there is no scientific proof that any of the prostate surgeries or treatments actually do extend a man's life. In fact, the Prostate Patient Outcomes Research Team has determined that a sixty-year-old man with moderately aggressive cancer, an excellent doctor, and surgery with minimal complications should live another seventeen years. But if the same man opts for "watchful waiting," he would probably live another sixteen years without the discomfort, risks, or complications of surgery.

The May 1993 issue of the *Journal of the American Medical Association* carried articles comparing the outcomes (adjusted for quality of life) of prostate cancer patients treated with radical prostatectomy, radiation, and "watchful waiting."[5] The authors of one article concluded that "we could find no study or group of studies in the medical literature that definitely supports the benefit of either treatment (surgery or radiation) over watchful waiting." The second article was an editorial written by the renowned Willet W. Whitmore, Jr., of the Memorial Sloan-Kettering Cancer Center in New York. Dr. Whitmore was intrigued by the question "What happens if you leave them alone?" He reviewed the histories of seventy-five men with stage B1, B2, and B3 cancers of the prostate. Forty-six of the patients eventually had some treatment (including radiation, surgery, and hormones). Dr. Whitmore found that after twenty or more years, there was very little difference in survival time between those treated and those who were not treated, in terms of whose cancers did not progress. These and other studies are not conclusive, but they give us food for thought.

"Watchful waiting" is a significant approach to prostate cancer. You may want to discuss this with your physician.

7

Alternative Approaches to Treating the Prostate

A fascinating study released in 1993 showed that Americans have a great deal of faith in alternative medicine. On the other hand, perhaps the study shows that we are losing faith in standard Western medicine. Whatever the case may be, we're turning to alternative forms of healing in greater numbers than ever before. And we're spending more money out-of-pocket for uninsured alternative health than we spend out-of-pocket for traditional medicine. (Much more is actually spent in standard medicine than on alternative approaches, but the bulk of the cost is covered by insurance.)

Perhaps part of the appeal of alternative therapies is that for the most part, they are not nearly as toxic or potentially dangerous as are the powerful drugs, radiation, chemotherapy, surgeries, and other standard treatments. The philosophy behind many of the alternative approaches is attractive as well: Help the body heal itself, rather than employing the standard idea of destroying the germs. Unfortunately, not all alternative therapies are safe and effective.

The alternative therapies discussed in this chapter are just a few of the many available. They are not meant to be a true sampling of all that is available; rather, they provide a brief look at some other approaches.

I am not necessarily recommending or endorsing any of these therapies. The information on alternative therapies presented in this chapter is provided for your information only. It is not intended to be medical advice. If you have a disease or any other condition, I urge you to see your physician, who will frequently work with alternative therapists, because the basic aim is to help the patient.

123

ALTERNATIVE APPROACHES TO
TREATING INFECTIONS AND BPH

"Anti-Beer"

Prolactin is a hormone that encourages the prostate to take in more testosterone and convert it to DHT. (It's the DHT that actually stimulates the prostatic overgrowth of BPH.) Some researchers feel that an ingredient (or a combination of ingredients) found in beer stimulates the pituitary gland to release more prolactin. Thus, avoiding beer has been proposed as a simple, nontoxic way of realigning body chemistry and reducing the symptoms of BPH.

Electric C

Electric C is a combination of vitamin C and electrolytes that has been shown to have a beneficial effect on the prostate, as well as on general health.

Hydrotherapy

The ancient treatment called hydrotherapy is the use of hot water, cold water, ice, or steam to treat disease and improve overall health. In the treatment of BPH, patients typically use a small tub called a sitz bath, in which the buttocks and lower belly are immersed in the water. A warm bath (up to 99°F) is used for acute prostatitis; a hot bath (up to 115°F) is used to open urinary passageways for patients with nonacute prostatitis; and a cold bath (between 55° and 75°F) following a warm or hot bath is used for general health benefits once the prostate problem has been cured. Contrast baths, with alternating hot and cold water, may be used to improve muscle tone and circulation in the pelvic area.

Plant Products

Various plant products have been found to be helpful in reducing prostate swelling, alleviating the pain, and reducing certain other symptoms. These natural health aids include Prostat, *Pygeum africanum*, *Equisetum arvense*, *Hydrangea arborescens*, *Serenoa serrulata*, and saw palmetto.

Prostat

Prostat contains an extract from pollen that has been used to treat BPH in Europe and Japan for years. In European studies of chronic prostatitis, 78 percent of men have had a favorable response to Prostat alone. Prostates enlarge when testosterone is converted into DHT within the prostate. Prostat shrinks the prostate by occupying the DHT receptors, locking out testosterone. Thus DHT cannot be made, and the prostate shrinks. The man's overall testosterone supply is left undisturbed; only the testosterone by-product in the prostate is affected. European and American studies are quite promising: Prostat relieves some of the symptoms of prostate problems, and shrinks the enlarged prostate. It is nontoxic and seems to be well tolerated. The product is completely hypoallergenic.

A study reported in the *British Journal of Urology*[1] compared Prostat (called Cernilton in Europe) to a placebo in a double-blind study of sixty men with urinary difficulties due to BPH. Following the six-month study, the authors concluded that Prostat "has a beneficial effect in BPH and may have a place in the treatment of patients with mild or moderate symptoms of outflow obstruction."

Another study[2] looked at the effects of the pollen extract on ninety men, ages 19 to 90, suffering from prostatitis and prostatodynia. The researchers found it to be "effective in the treatment of patients with chronic nonbacterial prostatitis and prostatodynia." However, it did not help those with complicating factors, such as strictures in the urethra or calcification of the prostate.

Prostat is manufactured by Pharmacia Allergon and distributed in the United States by Horizon Crest, Inc. (I am the principal United States investigator for Prostat. The results are remarkable; some 80 percent of those studied show good progress.)

Pygeum africanum

Pygeum africanum comes from an African evergreen tree and has a long history of use for urinary tract difficulties. Although only recently available in the United States, it has been studied for over twenty years. Controlled, double-blind studies have shown *Pygeum* to be very helpful in reducing prostate inflammation and symptoms of prostatitis. It has been used for prostate problems in Europe for some time.

Equisetum arvense

Researchers have noted that *Equisetum* helps to reduce prostatic inflammation and its attendant symptoms.

Hydrangea arborescens

Often used in conjunction with *Equisetum arvense, Hydrangea* helps reduce inflamed and enlarged prostates.

Serenoa serrulata

Berries of this American dwarf palm were part of the regular diet for some American Indians. In the nineteenth century, *Serenoa* was noted for its toning effects on the male reproductive system. It is felt that *Serenoa* blocks the formation of DHT, as well as the ability of DHT to bind to receptor cells in the prostate. *Serenoa* has been shown to increase urinary flow rate and to reduce the mean residual volume (what's left in the bladder after urination).

Saw palmetto

Extracted from a palm tree native to the Atlantic coast and the West Indies, saw palmetto (*Serenoa reopens*) has long been used to rejuvenate the man with prostate problems or flagging sexuality. It is felt that saw palmetto's beneficial effects on the prostate are due to its ability to inhibit DHT, thus helping to keep the prostate at its normal size.

Reflexology

Reflexology treats ailments by massaging certain areas of the feet or hands. The art goes back at least 5,000 years to the Chinese, and it was used by some Egyptians as far back as 3000 B.C.

According to reflexologists, the body is divided into many zones running up and down or across the body. The kidney is treated, for example, by locating it within the "gridwork," then treating (massaging) the corresponding area on the feet and hands. Although no one knows exactly why reflexology works, some of the theories that have been advanced for the success of the therapy include the following: It improves blood circulation; it stimulates the nervous system; it realigns energy systems within the body; it stimulates acupuncture points; it encourages the drainage of lymph fluid; and it removes crystal deposits of calcium at the end of the nerves in the feet. Overall, the attempt in reflexology is to balance the body, helping it to heal itself.

To treat prostate problems associated with infection and enlargement, the reflexologist will massage foot points corresponding to the prostate, the pituitary gland, the thyroid gland, the adrenal glands, the lymph system, the ureters, and the kidneys. The foot points corresponding to the urinary system are found on the bottom half of the right sole, on the arch side of the foot. In the hands, the prostate point is slightly below the thumb, on the edge of the hand.

SOME ALTERNATIVE HEALING PHILOSOPHIES

Western medicine is not the only complete system of healing with theories on the causes and cures of diseases and a black bag filled with medicines. There are other complete healing systems, including Ayurveda medicine, homeopathy, and Oriental medicine. Let's take a look at the three approaches, bearing in mind that the discussions that follow are very general, and are meant for educational purposes only.

Ayurveda Medicine

Ayurveda is an ancient medical system from India based on the principle that the mind and body are one, so the body cannot be well if the mind is troubled. Only recently introduced to the United States, Ayurveda is a holistic healing system that uses diet, massage, detoxification, herbal remedies, and breathing exercises to treat ailments.

According to Ayurveda philosophy, there are many possible causes of cancer, including a lack of purpose in life, a sedentary lifestyle, environmental toxins, and devitalized foods. It is thought that the cancer itself results from physical, emotional, and spiritual imbalances.

The three-stage treatment for cancer attempts to detoxify, balance, and rebuild the body through diet, herbs, meditation, spiritual and emotional therapy, and cleansing. Yoga, the chanting of mantras, and gem therapy to enhance the body's aura may also be used.

Scripps Institute in La Jolla, California, has recently opened a unit where Ayurveda medicine will be practiced, in addition to other modalities.

Homeopathy

Homeopathy was developed in the late 1700s by Samuel Hahnemann, a German physician. Unlike standard Western medicine, practitioners of homeopathy believe that "like cures like." In other words, a person with disease A can be cured by being administered a tiny dose of a substance that causes the symptoms of disease A in a healthy person. This principle is very similar to that underlying vaccines (a little bit of a germ helps the immune system fight off a full-fledged invasion of the same germ).

Whereas standard medicine looks upon symptoms as terrible things to be stamped out, homeopathy views symptoms as proper adaptations of the body to a problem. Symptoms come about because the body is trying to heal itself. Thus, instead of using powerful drugs to eliminate the symptoms, homeopathy attempts to help the body heal itself. The homeopathic doctor will use a small dose of a highly diluted homeopathic medicine to stimulate the body's natural healing processes.

The homeopath expects symptoms to be cured in the reverse order in which they appeared, and possibly to get worse before they get better. However, the patient should feel better overall (in spite of the temporary worsening of symptoms) because the body is stronger. Here are some of the homeopathic medicines that might be used for prostatitis (inflammation of the prostate).

Staphysagria: For urinary streams that stop and start, and for burning.

Pulsatilla: For pain after urinating, and certain penile discharges.

Kali bichromium: For severe prostate pain worsened by movement, burning after urination, and certain penile discharges.

Causticum: For urinary leakage when coughing, sneezing, or laughing, for pain following urination, and for retention of urine following surgery.

Sabal serrulata: For frequent urination and pain in the perineal area.

These or other homeopathic medicines may be given two to three times daily for several days, then stopped as soon as the symptoms improve. The medicines are given one at a time, not in a group.

Oriental Medicine

According to the theory of Oriental medicine,[3] prostate problems are caused by weakness or other difficulties in the kidney, spleen, or liver meridians. (There are twelve meridians, or invisible energy pathways, in the body.) Prostate problems may be caused by a weakness in the kidney meridian, by a dampness in the spleen meridian, by a blockage in the liver meridian, or by any combination of the three.

According to Oriental medicine, all prostate conditions, ranging from an infection to cancer, are due to problems with one or more of the three pertinent meridians. A greater problem with the meridian(s) means a more severe illness. Thus, all treatment aims to build up the kidney meridian, dry up the dampness in the spleen meridian, and/or remove the blockage in the liver meridian. The more severe the problem, the stronger, more stringent, or longer the treatment, but the basic principles will remain the same unless there is an actual growth (such as a tumor), which will then require specific herbs to break it up.

There are genetic, dietary, emotional, and other factors contributing to problems with the meridians. The kidney meridian, for example, may be weakened through a lifetime of stress. The liver meridian may be harmed if one is an alcoholic.

The treatment for prostate problems is highly individual, and it depends upon the individual's specific problems, overall health, and the type of doctor of Oriental medicine who is consulted. In general, however, treatment consists of acupuncture, Chinese herbal combinations, emotional changes, and diet to eliminate problems with the affected meridians.

1. Depending upon the specific doctor, patient, and meridian imbalance, acupuncture involves the placing of needles in and around the ankles, and in and around the lower stomach (between the belly button and the pubic area).
2. Some of the herbs that may be used include a genthinna combination (used mainly for the liver meridian) and a lotus seed combination (which works mainly with the kidney), as well as polyporus and dianthus formulas.
3. The dietary changes suggested would depend upon the meridians involved. If it is the liver meridian, fats, fried foods, and sugars would be eliminated. If the kidney meridian is afflicted, caffeine, sugar, and salt would be eliminated. If the spleen meridian is involved, the patient must eliminate all foods that cause dampness, including all dairy products, sugar, and fatty foods.

The course of treatment is typically twice a week for ten weeks. Treatment usually stops for about a month to allow for evaluation, then continues with additional ten-week courses as necessary. If the problem is relatively minor, the patient may be asked to come for treatment only once a week during a single, ten-week course.

Oriental medicine treats the person and the imbalance more than a specific problem. Thus, a difficulty with the prostate is felt to be only the "tip of the iceberg," so the Oriental doctor aims to restore the entire person to full physical and emotional health.

SOME ALTERNATIVE APPROACHES TO TREATING CANCER

Among the numerous alternative approaches to dealing with cancer, many are outlawed in the United States. This section discusses some alternative treatments in general, and not specifically for prostate cancer.

This very brief survey of alternative approaches is presented for educational purposes only—to make you aware of the range of alternatives that have been proposed. I am not recommending that you use any of these approaches to diagnose or treat yourself, or anyone else. If you have cancer or any other disease, I urge you to see your physician.

Antineoplaston Therapy

This approach deviates from modern medicine by arguing that a system of naturally occurring peptides and amino acid derivatives called antineoplastons—rather than the immune system—is responsible for controlling cancer. Proponents of antineoplaston therapy feel that these antineoplastons are like teachers who instruct errant (cancerous) cells how to behave themselves.

It's felt that the blood of cancer patients contains only 2 to 3 percent of the antineoplastons that it should; therefore, therapy consists of putting the antineoplastons back into the bloodstream, either orally or intravenously. Dr. Stanislaw Burzynski, of the Burzynski Research Institute in Houston, says that he has had very good success in treating some 2,000 patients, most with advanced cancer.

Burton's Immune Augmentative Therapy

This immune system-boosting therapy is meant to help control cancer by strengthening the body's natural defenses. Four blood proteins are used to treat the patient, the idea being that these four components are out of balance in the cancer patient. Treatment consists of analyzing the patient's blood daily, or twice daily, then giving injections of the appropriate proteins in order to bring the vital four proteins into the proper balance. Once patients have left the treatment center, they continue to self-administer the injections for as long as is necessary. Burton's immune augmentative therapy is not practiced in the United States, but there is an immune augmentative center in the Grand Bahamas.

Chaparral

A tea made from a desert shrub called chaparral has been used to treat cancer and other diseases for many years. Back in the 1940s, researchers at the University of Minnesota identified NDGA (nordihydroguaiaretic acid) as the active ingredient in chaparral that fights off cancer cells, viruses, bacteria, and fungi.

It is felt that NDGA attacks cancer in at least two ways: It slows the transport of electrons within the cancer cells' mitochondria (the little "energy factories" that power the cells). Lacking energy, cancer cells die. Studies suggest that NDGA also prevents enzymes from breaking down sugars and carbohydrates. Since cancer cells must ferment sugar in order to continue growing and multiplying, NDGA can "starve" the dangerous cells to death.

The FDA is investigating the use of chaparral, suspecting that it may be involved in a number of cases of toxic hepatitis. A hold has been put on chaparral until the investigation is completed.

Chelation Therapy

Also used to treat heart disease, chelation consists of injecting a chelating (binding) agent into the bloodstream. A substance called EDTA (ethylene diamine tetraacetic acid) is typically infused into the body intravenously (IV) as the chelating agent. (Various vitamins or other substances may be added to the chelation fluid.) The chelating agent acts like a "claw," grabbing up toxic heavy metals and binding to them. Trussed up, so to speak, by the chelating agent, the toxic substance is rendered harmless and passed out of the body in the urine.

No one knows exactly how chelation therapy may defeat cancer. One theory is that chelation binds up and helps to eliminate lead, mercury, and other potentially cancer-causing substances from the body. Others feel that chelation improves the overall circulation, making more oxygen available to body cells. Since cancer grows better in the absence of oxygen, improving the circulation may slow cancer growth. Still another theory is that the EDTA and other substances used in chelation may destroy the protein covering that protects cancer cells from the body's immune system.

Gerson Therapy

Devised by Max Gerson, M.D., this therapy is based on the idea that cancer cannot occur until the liver, pancreas, immune system, and other parts of bodily systems have weakened. According to Gerson, cancer is caused by faulty body metabolism, which is in turn the result of exposure to air and water pollution, pesticides, chemicals, and other toxins. Gerson therapy, thus, aims to detoxify the body.

To help flush toxins from the body, patients are put on a low-fat, salt-free diet based on fresh, organically grown fruits and vegetables. Patients are also required to drink thirteen glasses of fresh-squeezed juice every day. Supplements include thyroid extract, liver extract, niacin, and pancreatic enzyme.

The detoxification process is aided by coffee enemas, which are self-administered several times a day. It is felt that the caffeine stimulates the liver, increases the flow of bile, and opens up the bile ducts, all of which helps the liver to excrete toxic by-products of the tumor. Castor oil, taken by mouth or enema, is sometimes prescribed to assist in the detoxification.

Livingston Therapy

Acting on the belief that cancer is caused by bacteria, Livingston therapy attempts to combat cancer by supporting the immune system. Back in the 1940s, Dr. Virginia Livingston discovered what she felt was a form-changing organism that caused most cancers. She named the organism Progenitor cryptocides, which means "hidden, ancestral killer." Dr. Livingston believed that Progenitor cryptocides is naturally present in the human body, but is kept under control by the immune system. When stress, environmental toxins, poor diet, or other factors weaken the immune system, however, the cancer-causing bacteria "break loose" and cause cancer.

The Livingston therapy includes antibiotics, a vegetarian diet, gamma globulin, and vitamin and mineral supplements. A special vaccine, prepared specifically for each patient from a sample of his own bacteria, is also given. A vaccine of a weakened tuberculin vaccine called BCG (bacillus Calmette-Guerin) or other vaccines may also be given.

The therapy is used at the Livingston Foundation Medical Center in San Diego.

Macrobiotics

As explained by Michio Kushi, a leader in macrobiotics, the therapy *does not* consist of an all-brown-rice diet. Rather, macrobiotics is a way of life that includes a low-fat, high-fiber diet rich in complex carbohydrates. About half of the macrobiotic diet consists of whole grains; another quarter or third consists of vegetables; and the rest consists of sea vegetables, beans, soups, and occasional fish, nuts, seeds, fruits, and condiments. Foods that have been highly processed, treated with chemicals, or cooked with electricity are avoided, as are highly salted foods.

The miso soup, shiitake mushrooms, kelp, cruciferous vegetables (such as broccoli and cabbage), seaweed, and other components of the macrobiotic diet have been shown to slow the growth of cancer. The fact that the diet is low in fat and additives is also helpful in fighting cancer.

The full macrobiotic approach includes a positive mental outlook, maintaining strong personal relationships with friends and family, chewing the food well, plentiful exercise, the wearing of natural fabrics, and the use of natural cooking utensils. Chemical fumes, microwave ovens, and excessive television watching are avoided.

Shark Cartilage

The fact that sharks don't seem to get cancer has intrigued scientists for years. During a ten-year study at the Mote Marine Laboratory in Sarasota, Florida, sharks were deliberately exposed to high doses of carcinogens, yet they apparently did not develop any tumors.

Medical researchers know that tumors depend upon the growth of new blood vessels both to nourish them and to carry away wastes. They also know that a certain substance in cartilage slows or stops the growth of tumors in animals by inhibiting the growth of new blood vessels. Since sharks' skeletons are made entirely of cartilage (not bone), and sharks don't seem to get cancer, could this substance in cartilage that slows the growth of new blood vessels be the reason that sharks are almost entirely cancer-free?

In 1988, Dr. Ghanem Atassi of the Institut Jules Bordet in Belgium grafted human skin cancer (melanoma) onto forty mice. Half of the mice were given daily doses of shark cartilage, while the other half were left untreated. In three weeks, tumors in the untreated mice had doubled in size. But in those mice that had received shark cartilage, the tumors had actually decreased in size. Researchers worldwide are experimenting with shark cartilage as a treatment for cancer in humans, and early results have shown promise.

CONCLUSION

This brief presentation gives you an idea of the scope of alternative therapies that are available. In these first seven chapters, we've talked about the various prostate problems, their diagnoses, and treatment. But what should *you* do if you receive the unhappy diagnosis of prostate cancer? How do you sort through the reams of study and the often-conflicting advice? Chapter 8 presents an approach to decision making, should you be forced to respond to a diagnosis of cancer.

8

If the Diagnosis Is Cancer

Many years ago, my young son Steven and I were strolling through downtown Los Angeles when two men walking the opposite way, on the other side of the street, waved and called out: "Hey, there's the finger doctor!" When Steven asked me what they meant, I explained to him that each of these men—and all others who came to see me as patients—had had my gloved finger introduced into his rectum in an attempt to diagnose abnormalities of the prostate, especially cancer.

Understandably, many men do not like this examination. When I explain the benefits to them, however, almost all agree to undergo the procedure. One of the few who refused was a very "macho" fifty-two-year-old former marine drill sergeant who came to see me complaining of chest pain. When I began the prostate examination, he told me that "nobody is going to do that to me," and he kept insisting that there was no need for me to examine any part of his body except his chest.

I had been taught that a good specialist in internal medicine examines a patient completely, from head to toe. I explained to the man that being able to perform a complete examination would help me to make an accurate diagnosis. And I added that sometimes I could pick up a suspicious condition in the earliest stages, when it would be most easily treated. He still refused. It wasn't until the end of the physical examination that he said that I should do the digital rectal examination. His voice was less powerful and he looked away as he gave me the permission.

As soon as my finger touched his rock-hard, ridged prostate I knew that something was wrong. The patient knew it, too. He later confessed that he knew that "there was something seriously wrong in there, somewhere," but had been afraid to find out what it was. Complaining of chest pain was a ruse, an excuse to get him into a doctor's office, where he would deny any prostate problem but subconsciously hope that it would be found. We quickly learned that the cancer had engulfed much of his prostate and had begun spreading beyond. Although the statistics told us that he had many months, and perhaps years, of life ahead, this man seemed to crumble when he got the news. Despite the best efforts of many specialists, he worsened rapidly and quickly died.

As a doctor with forty years of experience in treating critically ill patients, I've seen this scenario often. For many people, the diagnosis of cancer is as deadly as the disease itself. Absolutely petrified by the thought of cancer, many seem to "die of fear." I understand why people are terrified by cancer—it can be an ugly disease. But it doesn't have to be. *I'm writing this chapter to tell you that the diagnosis of prostate cancer is most likely* not *a death sentence, and that the odds are that, with such a diagnosis, you will have many, many years of life ahead of you. As we have discussed and you'll see again, otherwise healthy men whose cancer is confined to their prostates will probably die of some other disease late in life, never even knowing that they had this cancer.*

A Growing Concern

According to the American Cancer Society, approximately 200,000 American men will be diagnosed with prostate cancer this year. Black men are significantly more at risk than are white men, although we don't know exactly why.

The number of cases of prostate cancer rose by 50 percent between 1980 and 1990, but don't be alarmed. This increase is apparently mostly due to the fact that we're better at finding it than we used to be. And as more sensitive tests are devised, we can expect to see the numbers of *detected* prostate cancers rise. (As far as we know, the number of *actual* prostate cancers may be holding steady. In other words, there may always have been large numbers of prostate cancer, but we didn't know it because the cancers caused few or no symptoms.)

Although prostate cancer is the cancer that American men get the most, it's only the #2 killer cancer. (Lung cancer is the deadliest. There were over 100,000 detected cases of lung cancer in 1994, and over 94,000 deaths.) Indeed, many men die *with* prostate cancer, but not *because* of it. Still, some 38,000 men died of the disease in 1995— and the odds of dying from the cancer have increased in the past decades. In 1958–1960, 20.5 out of every 100,000 men died of

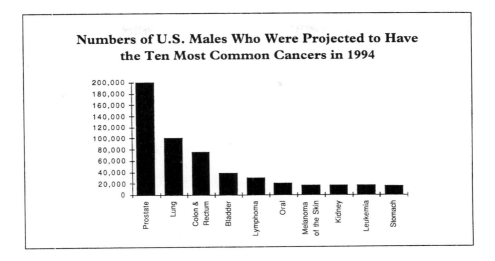

Numbers of U.S. Males Who Were Projected to Have the Ten Most Common Cancers in 1994

prostate cancer. In 1988–1990, the death rate had risen to 25.3 deaths per 100,000.

Having been perhaps alarmist with the numbers, let me again be reassuring by pointing out that heart disease and lung cancer are much larger problems for men than prostate cancer. Furthermore, having this cancer hardly means having to face death. We tend to get it in fairly high numbers, but somehow we learn to live with it.

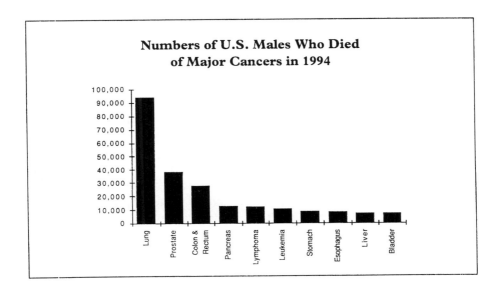

Numbers of U.S. Males Who Died of Major Cancers in 1994

The Dollars and Cents of Prostate Cancer

Exact figures are hard to come by, but it is estimated that prostate cancer costs us about $4 billion a year. About $2 billion goes for hospital and doctor bills, $200 million for prescription medicines, $200 million for nursing home care, and close to $1.5 billion is eaten up by the indirect costs of lost work productivity and wages as well as lost experience.

Despite the rapid increase in the number of diagnosed prostate cancer cases, the amount of money spent researching prostate cancer is low compared to other diseases. Federal funding amounts to approximately $1,400 for every new case of breast cancer, close to $550 for every new case of lung cancer, just shy of $500 for every new case of colorectal cancer, and only $250 for each new case of prostate cancer. This is not to suggest that we take money away from the researching of any of the other cancers. Rather, we should see more money spent studying all diseases.

ONE DISEASE, MANY FACETS

To the medical/scientific community, cancer has many meanings. Cancer is a tumor. Cancer is a malignancy. Cancer is a carcinoma, a sarcoma, a leukemia. Cancer is Hodgkin's disease, it is a mesothelioma, it is an adrenocarcinoma, it is a bronchogenic/carcinoma, it is a retinoblastoma. Cancer is a disease caused by radiation, free radicals, oxidation, viruses, smoking, overexposure to the sun, certain chemicals, and genetic errors. Cancer is related to a high-fat diet (especially to a diet high in animal protein and fat). Cancer can be slow; it can be fast. Cancer can be tolerated for quite some time, or it can attack with deadly swiftness. Cancer is many things, yet stripped to the essentials it is just this: the unregulated growth of previously normal body cells, the dangerous proliferation of a cell gone bad. One cell divides into two, the two become four, the four eight, the eight sixteen, the sixteen thirty-two, and on and on. As the renegade cells grow, they "forget" the rules of cooperation that body cells live by. They forget that they're supposed to take in certain limited amounts of nutrients, and to perform certain functions. They forget that they're but small parts of a whole, working for the good of the entire body.

The human body is a marvelous structure. Working with relatively few materials, the body builds organs, systems, and structures, each separate and unique yet interlocking, each with unique identities.

Body cells are divided by type, even within organs, each type having specific functions. Cells in the pituitary gland produce hormones for "long distance" communication. Cells of the heart contract in rhythm with their fellows. Each red blood cell is part of the massive fleet of blood-borne "buses" that carry oxygen to and fro. A liver cell is a liver cell; it cannot be a muscle cell. Every cell contributes by performing its specific function. Some have likened body cells to citizens in some ideal paradise, each one working for the benefit of the whole, taking back only what it needs.

Despite their differences, all cells have common characteristics, for each is born of the same strand of genetic material. Cancer cells, too, have a common characteristic, a goal: They're driven to grow. Somehow they come to ignore the rules that tell all cells to cooperate in a civilized manner. Instead, they revert to a wild and primitive stage, interested only in feeding and growing.

"Double Life"

Scientists speak of the half-life of radioactive substances as a way of describing how long they will remain dangerous. I like to think of the "double life" of cancer cells as a way of measuring their voracious growth. A single cancerous cell only has to double roughly thirty times before it's big (about ½ inch). These thirty doublings turn a single cancer cell into over a billion cells. With each doubling, there are greedy, unrestrained cells trampling upon nearby "good" cells. Your body's immune system is continually reining in and destroying the cancerous growth. If your immune system is successful, you'll probably never know that you had cancer. But if the cancer is too strong, or if your immune system is too weak, the cancer will eventually take over.

After the first thirty doublings, only another ten are needed to turn ½ inch of cancer into 2.2 pounds of cancer—usually enough to kill. Some cancers, such as stomach carcinoma, grow rapidly. Others, including cancer of the prostate and thyroid, may grow slowly, often going unnoticed for years.

"STAGING" THE CANCER

A frightened and confused man called me at the office one day, practically spitting out his words:

> *I went to my doctor and he told me I had cancer. When I asked him how bad it was he said it was a 'B-plus,' and then he left the room! I liked getting B-pluses on my tests in school because that was above average, but I don't know if an above-average cancer is good or bad. In other words,* what the hell was my doctor talking about?

Like a cold or a case of pneumonia, cancer can be relatively mild or fatally severe. To help describe how mild or severe we believe a cancer to be, physicians have come up with a means of "staging" cancer, which simply means to describe the stage to which the cancer has progressed (similar to the stages of life we humans experience).

This man's doctor was using the "A, B, C" system of staging the cancer that is favored by the National Cancer Institute:

Stage A—Microscopic cancer cells can be found in prostate tissue examined in a laboratory. The cancer cannot be seen with the naked eye, cannot be felt upon digital rectal examination, and has produced no symptoms. In fact, it's only found accidently when doctors are operating for other reasons (such as BPH) and send prostate tissue to the laboratory for routine examination.

> *Stage A1*—The microscopic cancer cells are found only in one area of the prostate.

> *Stage A2*—The microscopic cancer cells are found in more than one area of the prostate.

Stage B—The doctor can feel a tumor in the prostate during a digital rectal examination, but the cancer is confined to the prostate.

Stage C—Although still in the prostate, the cancer has pushed through the covering of the prostate and grown into nearby tissue. The seminal vesicles or bladder neck may have been invaded by the cancer.

Stage D—The cancer has extended beyond the prostate, spreading to more distant lymph nodes, organs, or tissues.

> *Stage D1*—The cancer has spread to lymph nodes near the prostate.

Stage D2—The cancer has spread to lymph nodes far away from the prostate, or has spread to the bone, liver, lungs, or other parts of the body.

Recurrent—Although it was already treated and supposedly eliminated, the cancer has returned to the prostate or to another part of the body.

There are variations of this standard A, B, C staging system, but the basic idea is that if you do have cancer, an "A" is most preferred. The American Cancer Society has devised another, easy-to-understand system of describing prostate cancer:[1]

Very Early—In this stage, the cancer is confined to the prostate gland and cannot be felt during a rectal examination. Rather, a case such as this is detected when a patient has surgery for what was thought to be benign prostate disease, but whose biopsy reveals cancer. In many cases, patients with very early cancers receive no additional treatment at that time but are advised to return for follow-ups at regular intervals.

Localized—These cancers are confined to the prostate gland but are large enough to be palpated during a rectal examination.

Regionalized—These tumors have spread into the tissues immediately surrounding the prostate gland.

Advanced—Tumors have spread to the lymph nodes in the pelvis or beyond, or to other bodily structures, usually the bones.

Yet another system for staging cancer is called the TNM system, which focuses on the anatomy of a tumor by looking at (1) the Tumor, (2) the lymph Nodes of the region, and (3) the Metastasis.

In the T-stage, the cancer hasn't spread yet. It's a single tumor, such as a lump in the breast. If the surgeons can remove the entire tumor, chances for complete recovery are excellent.

Next is the N-stage. No longer contained, the tumor has begun to spread to the local lymph glands, which, packed with immune cells, try to halt the cancer. As the battle rages, the lymph glands become enlarged. If the cancer cells win the battle, they fill the swollen lymph nodes and start leaking out to other parts of the body. In procedures such as prostatectomy, surgeons often remove the lymph glands and send them to the laboratory for examination, to determine whether the cancer has spread to the lymph glands.

The M-stage is the most dangerous, for now there is a metastasis, a cancer that has spread to distant parts of the body. Even if the main tumor is removed, there is danger from each of the daughter cells.

Here's a TNM classification system specifically designed for prostate cancer:[2]

T: The Primary Tumor

TX — Tumor cannot be assessed
T0 — No evidence of tumor
T1 — Tumor is not clinically apparent, is not palpable, cannot be visualized (seen) with imaging devices
T2 — Tumor is confined to the prostate
T3 — Tumor has broken through the prostatic capsule
T4 — Tumor has invaded or fixed itself to adjacent tissue (other than the seminal vesicles)

N: The Lymph Nodes

NX — Cannot be assessed
N0 — No evidence of spread to regional lymph nodes
N1 — Spread to a single lymph node
N2 — Larger spread to a single lymph node, or to more than one node
N3 — Spread to a regional lymph node

M: The Metastasis

MX — Cannot be assessed
M0 — No evidence that the cancer has spread to distant areas
M1 — The cancer has spread to distant areas

All three of these cancer-staging systems (A-D, Early-Advanced and TNM) are useful tools for describing what a particular cancer is doing inside the body. If your doctor has yet another staging system, insist that he or she describe it to you in detail.

"GRADING" THE CANCER: THE GLEASON SCALE

Staging systems help you and your doctor to understand where the cancer is and how far it has spread. Simply knowing where it is, however, does not tell us how dangerous it is likely to be. There have been patients whose cancers simply sat in place for many months, even years, apparently without growing any more dangerous. On the other hand, there are cancers that spread rapidly throughout a patient's body. That's why we need to know how likely it is that the cancer will continue to grow—how greedy it is, how malignant.

The Gleason scale, or Gleason grade, gives us some indication of how dangerous the cancer is likely to be. When the laboratory studies a tissue sample (taken during a biopsy or during an operation), the pathologist looks to see whether the cancer cells are well- or poorly differentiated (shaped). The cells are rated 1 to 5, with 1 meaning that the cells are well-differentiated, and 5 meaning that they are very poorly differentiated. The better the differentiation, the "safer" the cancer. Figure 8.1 shows an idealized picture of the five types of Gleason cells.

The laboratory will assign Gleason values to the various patterns it finds in the tissue sample, then add together the two most prominent patterns. Let's say your sample shows a lot of 1, a moderate amount of 2, and a tiny bit of 3 and 4. The laboratory would take the two most prominent patterns, 1 and 2, and add them together to give you a Gleason score of 3. If your tissue sample showed a lot of patterns 2 and 3, with smaller amounts of 1 and 4, the laboratory would add together 2 and 3 to get a Gleason score of 5.

Because the Gleason score is made up of two numbers ranging from 1 to 5, the lowest score you can have is 2, and the highest is 10. The lower your score, the better. Generally speaking, cancers with Gleason scores of 2 to 4 are considered to be well-differentiated, those with scores of 5 to 7 are moderately differentiated, and scores of 8 or above indicate a poorly differentiated cancer.

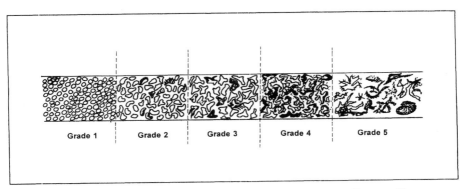

Grade 1   Grade 2   Grade 3   Grade 4   Grade 5

FIGURE 8.1 This highly stylized drawing shows cells with different Gleason ratings. *Illustration by R. C. F.*

Remember: The Gleason *patterns* grade tissue samples on a scale of 1 to 5. The two most prominent patterns are added together to give the Gleason *score*, which runs from 2 to 10.

"GRADING" THE CANCER: PLOIDY

A second system, informally called "ploidy," is also used to estimate just how dangerous (how aggressive) a cancer is likely to be. Ploidy refers to the number of complete chromosome sets in a cell. Tumor cells are labeled "diploid," "tetraploid," or "aneuploid" by the laboratory.

Unfortunately, there is not complete agreement upon what to do with the ploidy results. However, generally speaking, diploid cancers are considered somewhat less likely to be aggressive, and aneuploid cancers are thought to be more aggressive. Also, a cell's ploidy can change, so your physician may repeat the ploidy test over time.

WHAT CAUSES CANCER?

When I was eight, my five-year-old cousin was diagnosed as having cancer shortly after being kicked in the stomach. We all knew that the kick had caused the cancer. Now, thanks to scientific advances, we have a better understanding of the cancer process, although we have a lot more to learn.

As I mentioned in Chapter 1, two steps are required for a normal cell to become cancerous: initiation and activation. First, the cell's genetic instructions must be damaged or altered, initiating the cell. Then, days or years or decades later, the cell is activated. Among other things, the list of initiators and activators includes excess dietary fat, radiation, and various chemicals.

Although the specific causes of prostate cancer are unknown, we do know that growing older, being black, and eating a high-fat diet are all risk factors. Some studies have shown a relationship between increased risk of prostate cancer and having worked with or been exposed to the metal cadmium (used during welding, battery-making, and electroplating). Working in the rubber industry also seems to be associated with an increased risk. Having had a vasectomy has been associated with the disease by some experts, but others feel that there is no link. The cancer seems to run in families to some extent, but it's unclear if that's because of "cancer-prone" genes or because unhealthy habits are being passed from generation to generation. Prostate cancer is more common in North America and northwestern Europe, but it is rare in Central and South America, the Near East, and Africa.

IF THE DIAGNOSIS IS CANCER . . .

The most important thing to remember is that you always have options, no matter what the disease. You can decide to fight back, or you can choose to let nature take its course, no matter where it leads you. You may want to undergo the most difficult and painful of procedures, holding tight to even the smallest chance of success. Or you may opt for an alternative treatment. Whatever you do, make sure it's what *you* want to do. Don't let your doctors decide for you, or talk you into or out of anything. It's your health and your body, so it's your choice.

Step 1: Before You Do Anything Else . . .

First and foremost, make sure that the doctor overseeing your treatment is a very competent, very caring "general" doctor. Don't let a urologist—or a surgeon, or an oncologist (cancer specialist), or any other specialist—oversee your cancer treatment. Specialists tend to know everything there is to know about their fields of expertise, but not enough about patients as people.

For example, I've seen too many surgeons perform technically brilliant surgeries on people who should never have had them in the first place. Why are some surgeries unnecessary? There are many reasons. Sometimes the anticipated benefits are so small that they are not worth the risks. Sometimes the risks of surgery are greater than the possible benefits. Sometimes the patient doesn't need the surgery: A seventy-five-year-old man with no wife, no girlfriend, and absolutely no interest in sex probably doesn't need surgery to improve erectile function. The same seventy-five-year-old man with Stage A cancer of the prostate absolutely *does not* need surgical removal of the prostate, because the overwhelming odds are that he will die of other causes long before his cancer becomes dangerous. Yet, surgeons are trained to operate. When they see a problem, they tend to think of surgical solutions. These solutions may often be brilliant, but they are not always necessary, *and they are always risky, at best.*

Like surgeons, urologists tend to have limited perspectives. They are superb when it comes to dealing with urological problems, but they are not trained to deal with patients as people. Neither are oncologists.

If your diagnosis is cancer, do not agree to any invasive tests, treatments, medicines, or surgeries until you've consulted with a caring, competent general doctor (unless it's an emergency situation, in which case immediate action may be required). Unless it is an emergency, before you do anything else you should see your regular internist, general practitioner, family practitioner, or gerontologist (a doctor who specializes in helping the elderly). You may still need a surgeon, a urologist, and an oncologist, but insist that these talented specialists work under the direction of the caring general doctor who knows you well.

Put yourself at the head of your treatment team. Use your general doctor as an educator—a guide and an interpreter—who assists you in making choices and helps you to direct your helpers (the other doctors).

Step 2: Assess Yourself, Your Life

"I wouldn't say that getting cancer was a good thing, Dr. Fox," sixty-one-year-old Alan said with a little laugh. "But it did get me thinking about what was important to me. I thought I was going to die when they told me. But, you know, the first thought that came into my head was not that I wouldn't ever be company president, but that I wouldn't see my daughter's wedding. Wow! That made me rethink all my priorities. Enjoying my family shot up to number one on my list. Making president dropped way down. Since then, the last twenty years have been the best of my life.

The diagnosis of cancer is a turning point in many people's lives. The fear of death, or in some cases the knowledge that death is imminent, has a remarkable way of focusing and clarifying one's thoughts. For some people, the diagnosis is a kick in the stomach. For others, it's a call to action: There are doctors to see, treatments to undergo, strange medicines or vitamins to swallow. For some people, the diagnosis is a call to mend fences with friends and families, to redouble efforts to finish personal and business projects. For still others, the diagnosis is a release, "permission" to pass away.

One man, a seventy-three-year-old father of three and grandfather of ten, was perfectly content to die. Not that he was looking forward to death, but, as he said: "I've lived my life; I married a great gal; I raised my children; I held a steady job for fifty years. I've had great friends. I've gone through all the stages of life. If my time has come, so be it."

Another man, also seventy-three years old, kept saying that he refused to die "until that blankety-blank brother of mine dies first!"

If your diagnosis is cancer, you've come to a turning point, a great time to assess yourself and your life—who you are, what you want to achieve, how you want to be viewed by others, how you want to be remembered, whom you're angry at, whom you love, what you like most about life, what you would most like to change, and so on. Without being morbid or unduly alarmed, think about what would happen if you became too sick to work, if you were bedridden, or if you died. Consider all the possibilities, good, bad, and indifferent. To help my cancer patients assess their lives and determine their priorities, I give them a series of sentences to complete. There answers are not "right" or "wrong"; they simply serve to mirror one's attitudes and feelings.

Here's how a pleasant, fifty-six-year-old salesman completed the sentences:

I am — *a pretty nice guy, I do my best*

The most important things in life are — *family, work, and friends, in that order*

My goal in life is — *to raise my kids to follow the Golden Rule*

Others see me — *as a nice guy, maybe a bit of a pushover because I give in on a lot of things instead of throwing a fit*

The best thing in life is — *family*

The thing that bothers me most is — *injustice, especially to children*

If I could redo some part of my life I'd— *be smarter in picking my jobs*

I see my own death as — *the final curtain dropping on a great play*

If it would postpone my death, I'd — *right now, I'd do whatever it takes; surgery, radiation, chemicals. In another ten years or so, I'd just let the disease take its natural course.*

Right now, I feel— *ready to lick this cancer!*

Someday, I'd like my tombstone to say — *Here lies the father of four great kids*

This salesman enjoyed living. He knew what he wanted out of life, and how he wanted to live. When I told him that he had cancer, he took the news relatively calmly, focusing all his concern on his family. But he was willing to fight for his life, and so far, years later, he's still winning.

Here's how a thirty-five-year-old struggling television writer completed the sentences:

I am — the dishrag that directors, producers and actors abuse—the dregs

The most important things in life are — kissing butt so I can sell a script

My goal in life is — to make everyone who makes me miserable, just as miserable as I am—even more miserable

Others see me — as a doormat

The best thing in life is — winning, but I've forgotten what it feels like

The thing that bothers me most is — I'm not rich and powerful

If I could redo some part of my life I'd — be someone else

I see my own death as — something my enemies would like

If it would postpone my death, I'd — what's the point of trying?

Right now, I feel — helpless. What's the point of trying?

Someday, I'd like my tombstone to say — He got back at them

For a man so unhappy with life, he certainly was desperate to hang on to it. He cried when I gave him the unhappy diagnosis, saying over and over again, "It's just my luck to get shafted again." For him, the diagnosis was the final proof that his life was worthless, and that he was a complete failure. He made no efforts to cooperate with his oncologist, and died relatively soon.

Now hold the mirror to your own soul by completing the following sentences:

I am—

The most important things in life are—

My goal in life is—

Others see me—

The best thing in life is—

The thing that bothers me most is—

If I could redo some part of my life I'd—

I see my own death as—

If it would postpone my death, I'd—

Right now, I feel—

Someday, I'd like my tombstone to say—

Look carefully at your answers. What do they tell you about your-self? What are your priorities? Knowing that you may die sooner than anticipated, what do you want to do? What do you want to change about yourself? Do you want to hang on to life, or are you ready to give it up? Are you willing to fight the disease? To live with it? To surren-der? (These are not the only questions you should ask yourself if the diagnosis is cancer. Rather, they are a sampling of the kinds of issues that I review with my patients and suggest that they consider carefully.)

It's great to fight back. It's also appropriate, in certain cases, to let nature take its course. Whatever you do, make sure it's what *you* want to do, not what your doctors, your family, or others tell you is best for you.

Step 3: Gather Information

Having selected a good general doctor and examined yourself and your goals, gather as much information about yourself and your disease as possible. Give your doctor(s) the third degree. Ask them questions about the therapies, medicines, and surgeries that they recommend. *You have the right to know, and the doctor has the obligation to inform you.* Here are some of the many questions you should ask:

- Are you absolutely sure that I have cancer? What did you base your diagnosis on?
- What are the various treatments for my cancer? Which do you suggest? Why? What is the goal of this treatment (to eliminate the cancer entirely, to hold it back for a few years, to reduce pain)? Exactly what does the treatment consist of? How long will the treatment last?

- What are *all* the potential complications and side effects of the treatment, from the most common to the least common? What will you do to keep those complications and side effects to a minimum? What will you do should they become serious?
- How will the treatment affect my ability to work? To enjoy my hobbies? To take care of myself? How will it affect my mood and energy? My sexual life? My family?
- How will we know if the treatment is working? What happens if the treatment doesn't work as planned? What happens if it works, but my cancer later comes back?
- If you will be working with another doctor, who will be in charge of my treatment? How will you communicate with each other? Who will handle pain control, should I experience pain?
- Is there another treatment suitable for me? Why or why not? Please describe the alternative treatments, even if you do not endorse them.

No question is too silly or unimportant to ask. It's also helpful to ask your doctor for the names and telephone numbers of other patients who have undergone the treatment that is being recommended. Talk to those people. You'll get much of the same information from the patient's point of view, and will likely hear some things the doctors don't know about, or don't like to talk about.

After you've talked to your doctor(s), and to other men who have had various treatments, put your thoughts down on paper. Write down such information as:

1. I am _____ years old.
2. I am (married/single)_____ .
3. I have (number) _____ children.
4. Except for the cancer, my general health is _____ .
5. My cancer is stage _____ .
6. My Gleason score is _____ .
7. My ploidy is _____ .
8. My doctor says I can expect to live until age _____ .
9. I would like to live until age _____ .
10. My feelings about undergoing surgery are _____
    _____
    _____ .
11. My feelings about being radiated are _____
    _____
    _____ .

12. My feelings about taking hormones are _____
    _____
    _____ .

13. Generally speaking, I prefer (circle one) very conservative treatment, the latest treatment, alternative treatment.

14. I've discussed my cancer with (number) _____ doctors.

15. My doctor suggests the following treatment _____
    _____ ,

    which has these possible benefits _____
    _____
    _____

    and these possible side effects _____
    _____
    _____ .

    I think that the best part of this suggested treatment is _____
    _____
    _____ .

    The worst part is _____
    _____
    _____ .

    This treatment will keep me in the hospital for ____ days, off work
    for ____ days, in need of care or assistance for ____ days, and
    unable to perform my chores and hobbies for ____ days.

    The treatment costs $ _____ . My insurance will cover
    about $ _____ of that.

    The men I've spoken to who have already undergone this treatment tell me _____
    _____
    _____ .

    My impression of this treatment is _____
    _____ .

16. The doctor offering a *second opinion* suggests _____
    _____
    _____ ,

    which has these possible benefits _____
    _____

    and these possible side effects _____
    _____

I think that the best part of this suggested treatment is _____ .

_____

The worst part is _____ .

_____

This treatment will keep me in the hospital for ____ days, off work for ____ days, in need of care or assistance for ____ days, and unable to perform my chores and hobbies for ____ days.

The treatment costs $ _____ . My insurance will cover about $ _____ of that.

The men I've spoken to who have already undergone this treatment tell me _____

_____

_____ .

My impression of this treatment is _____

_____ .

NOTE: Use additional sheets of paper to record the information you receive from additional doctors, as well as your impressions of the treatments they suggest.

17. The thing I most want from my treatment is _____

_____ .

18. The thing I fear the most is _____

_____ .

19. Setting aside what the doctors have suggested, the treatment that makes the most sense to me is _____

_____ .

20. Before making a decision, I must learn more about _____

_____ .

21. Other pertinent information _____

_____

_____

_____ .

Writing out this information will help you to analyze both the suggested treatments and your own feelings.

Step 4: Lean On Your General Doctor, Direct the Others

Review all the medical and surgical options with your general doctor. Insist that he or she go over everything with you, repeating and re-explaining as much as necessary. Direct all the other physicians, surgeons, and anyone else involved to report their findings and recommendations to your general doctor. Do so gently but firmly, making it clear that while you trust them completely, you want one person to be the repository and conduit of information. (I've seen too many cases become disasters because no one was making sure that everyone was fully informed and cooperating. For various reasons, doctors communicate only in a limited way when left on their own.)

Step 5: Make Your Decision!

Whatever you decide—whether it is to fight like hell or go out with grace—make sure everyone knows your decision. But through it all, remember that you have the right to change your mind at any time.

CHOOSING THE BEST TREATMENT FOR YOUR PROSTATE CANCER

There are five main categories of treatment for cancer of the prostate: surgery, radiation, hormone therapy, chemotherapy, and "watchful waiting." The treatment that is best for you depends upon the stage your cancer has reached, as well as your attitudes toward both cancer and life. Remember that surgeons swear by surgery, radiation oncologists insist that radiation is the only way to go, and other specialists promote their own approaches. *Select the treatment plan that's best for* you, *not the one your specialist likes best.* (For more information on cancer, see the list of Cancer and Urologic Information Resources in the Appendix.)

We looked at medicines and surgeries for prostate cancer in Chapters 4 and 5. My own Healthy Prostate Program is presented in Chapters 11 and 12.

Should Men Be Screened for Prostate Cancer?

Many experts suggest that large numbers of men be screened for prostate cancer. Others argue that it's a waste of time and money, and may even hurt men. Here are the arguments for and against massive screening for prostate cancer.

In Favor of Screening

- The DRE can easily be performed as part of the routine physical examination, and the PSA can be added to the standard blood test at very little additional extra cost. Between them, the DRE and PSA can detect a large number of cancers before they spread.

- It is imperative that we detect prostate cancer *before* it spreads beyond the prostate, while it is still curable.

- The American Cancer Society and the American Urological Association recommend annual DREs and PSAs for all men fifty and older.

Against Screening

- The costs are quite high. Although adding a DRE to the standard physical examination costs next to nothing, not all men have annual physicals. Screening and treating every cancer will break the bank.

- We may find lots of cancer, but what's the point of subjecting men to harsh and possibly dangerous treatments if most of them will die without ever knowing they had prostate cancer?

- The screening tests will produce many "false positives," men who are told they have cancer when they don't. This will lead to unnecessary treatment and suffering.

- Even if we find cancers, current treatments aren't able to lengthen men's lives by very much.

- No major study comparing large-scale screening to nonscreening has shown that screening is beneficial.

My Opinion

Let's do the screening. What we save in health and happiness will make up for the cost. We'll also learn a lot about prostate cancer—its detection and progression.

IN ADDITION TO YOUR TREATMENT . . .

What follows is a general discussion of nutritional means to supplement your primary treatment for prostate cancer. Nutritional therapy should be considered an adjunct to treatment, but not as treatment by itself.

Although we don't know exactly why a person may get a particular cancer, studies have suggested that either a lack or an excess of certain dietary elements can play a role in the formation of cancer. Some feel that nutritional therapy may even be of benefit after diagnosis. Since there is no downside to using nutritional therapy in conjunction with other approaches, it is certainly worth considering.

We still don't fully understand what causes cells to become initiated and activated cancer cells, so we must look to all types of cancer in order to draw some tentative conclusions. Many studies have linked various types of cancer to eating a diet excessively high in fat, as well as to low levels of vitamin A, beta carotene (the plant form of vitamin A), vitamin C, vitamin E, the mineral selenium, and other nutrients.

Certain other studies have suggested that nutrients play a role in keeping the immune system strong. Since the immune system is our primary defense against all cancers, it pays to keep our "Department of Defense" as strong as possible, at all times. Even if cancer has struck, it pays to keep the immune system strong, for it continues to wage war against the disease. Here are a few of the reports pointing to the positive role nutrition plays in keeping the immune system strong.

Protein—A lack of protein can weaken the immune system.[3] This is not a problem for the average American, who consumes far more protein than needed on a daily basis.

Vitamin A—A lack of vitamin A reduces the ability of T cells and B cells to respond to invading organisms and other problems.[4] With a severe deficiency, the thymus and spleen can shrink. (The thymus and spleen are important "hangouts" for immune system cells.) In addition, the number of lymphocytes and leukocytes in the blood can fall (meaning that there are fewer cells available for battle).

Beta carotene—Beta carotene supplementation helps to stimulate the immune system's response to trouble, and may also help increase the number of the crucial helper T cells.[5]

The B-complex Family of Vitamins—Deficiencies of the B vitamins are associated with a decrease in the immune system's ability to fight invaders, both cell to cell and by producing antibodies.[6]

Vitamin C—A significant deficiency of C impairs the ability of the immune-system cells (phagocytes) to "eat" invading or offending organisms and cells.[7] A controlled study involving healthy students given 1,000 mg of C a day showed that C supplementation may strengthen the immune system.[8]

Vitamin E—A lack of vitamin E can harm the immune system in many ways, including a decrease in its ability to respond to danger by producing immunoglobulin, and a decrease in the ability of certain immune-system cells to multiply in the face of specific dangers. Supplementation with vitamin E may strengthen immune-system response to danger and may also increase the number of antibody-forming cells and enhance the cell-mediated responses.[9]

Copper—A lack of copper has been associated with increased infections and an impaired ability of immune-system cells to tackle problems.[10]

Iron—A deficiency may both impair the ability of the immune system to defeat bacteria and slow down the ability of certain immune-system cells to multiply in the face of danger. Even a relatively small (10 percent) decrease in dietary iron can weaken the immune system.[11]

Magnesium—Without sufficient amounts of the mineral magnesium, the immune system's ability to form antibodies is diminished, and the thymus can atrophy.[12]

Selenium—If selenium levels drop too far, the ability of certain immune-system cells to "absorb" invading organisms or to tackle other problems may be diminished, and the vital T cells may become obstructed and sluggish. If both selenium and vitamin E levels are low, cell-mediated immunity may be compromised.[13]

Zinc—A lack of the mineral zinc has been associated with immune-system weakness.[14]

This has been just a brief overview of the role of nutrients in supporting immune-system function. Optimal eating and a program supplementation will be discussed in Chapter 11. Even if you already have cancer, nutritional therapy can be a helpful supplement to your other treatment.

A QUICK NOTE ON VASECTOMY
AND PROSTATE CANCER

Many men have panicked after reading that vasectomies can cause prostate cancer. Having had vasectomies one, five, or fifteen years ago, they are now sure that the little pains in their groins mean that they have cancer. And they may have cause to worry, since some studies have linked vasectomies to prostate cancer.

A six-year, case-controlled study reviewed 614 patients with prostate cancer, as well as 2,588 patients in control groups who had other types of cancer. According to the researchers, having a vasectomy increased the risk of developing prostate cancer at all ages. More specifically, they found a 2.2 relative risk of developing the cancer in men who had had a vasectomy 13 to 18 years before (compared to a 1.7 relative risk for men who had not had the operation). The researchers felt that the risk of developing the cancer increased with the length of time since the vasectomy, although they cautioned that further study is necessary.[15]

Another study compared 220 men experiencing their first episodes of prostate cancer to 960 men with other kinds of cancer and to 571 without cancer. In this eleven-year study, those who had had a vasectomy had a 3.5 relative risk of developing prostate cancer compared to the cancer controls (men with other kinds of cancer), and a 5.3 relative risk compared to the noncancer controls. Unlike the above study, this one found no link between the length of time since vasectomy was performed and the development of prostate cancer.[16]

Like the authors of both of the above studies, I believe that more research is needed before we can say with certainty that vasectomies are or are not related to prostate cancer. In the meantime, if you've had a vasectomy and are concerned, help to keep your immune system strong by adopting the Healthy Prostate Program outlined in Chapter 11.

9

Dealing with the Serious Side Effects of Prostate Problems

The sobbing wife took me aside late one night at the hospital. Her husband's cancer had spread to his bones, and both husband and wife knew that he might suffer severe pain in the near future. "Harry can stand dying," she said. "But neither of us can stand to see him in bad pain. We don't want him to spend his last months suffering severely. Can't you do something?"

Like many others, Harry and his wife were more frightened by the prospect of terrible side effects, especially pain, than they were of the prostate cancer itself. For prostate patients, the three side effects men fear most are incontinence, impotence, and pain. Fortunately, there are ways to deal with these problems.

INCONTINENCE

Urinary incontinence (inability to hold your urine) is *not* a normal part of aging. We should all be able to control urination throughout life. Unfortunately, many prostate patients have mild to moderate urinary-control problems, while many of those who have had surgery find themselves wearing diapers. One of my patients, who had a total prostatectomy before he came to see me, angrily announced that he felt "like a water can with no stopper on the spout."

The brief discussion of incontinence that follows will introduce some of the problems as well as the solutions.

158

What Causes Incontinence?

As discussed in Chapter 1, muscles at the base of the bladder and right below the prostate help men to control their urine. Unfortunately, surgery and radiation can damage these urinary-control mechanisms. Other problems can cause incontinence, including a damaging growth left untouched by the surgeon's knife, urethral strictures, postoperative urinary tract infections, and some medicines.

We don't know exactly how many prostate patients develop incontinence, because the estimates vary considerably from study to study. We do know that the incontinence rate following radical prostatectomy is high. Estimates in the urological literature vary widely, with some researchers saying that only 2.5 percent of men wind up incontinent, and others saying that the actual incidence is well over 80 percent. Besides being messy and inconvenient, incontinence following prostatectomy may also be psychologically devastating for men who had absolutely no urinary problems before surgery.

Types of Incontinence

Although the result of incontinence is the same, it can be classified in several ways:

Stress incontinence

Losing urine when sneezing, laughing, or coughing, or when moving in certain ways. Men with stress incontinence may leak urine when they get out of a chair, get out of bed, move about, exercise, or walk, for example.

Urge incontinence

Losing urine as soon as the urge hits, before one can get to the bathroom. People with urge incontinence can't seem to get to the bathroom fast enough. They may have to go after drinking even small amounts of liquid.

Overflow incontinence

Feeling that the bladder is never really empty. Men with overflow incontinence often dribble urine throughout the day and night, spend a lot of time in the bathroom, pass only small amounts of urine at a time, and have a dribble rather than a flow of urine.

Your doctor may use blood tests, urinalysis, cystoscopy, or urodynamic testing if you complain of incontinence. A postvoid residual measurement (PVR) may also be recommended, which involves using ultrasound or a small tube placed in the bladder to measure how much urine remains in your bladder after you urinate. A stress test may also be used to see how much urine you lose when exercising, coughing, or performing other chores.

Incontinence Treatments

The treatment for incontinence depends upon the type (the cause). Once the type has been established, treatment may begin, including:

Collecting the fluid

Urine is collected immediately by devices such as diapers, small-capacity collectors that fit right over the penis, and clamps that close off the penis, temporarily preventing leakage. These are not cures for incontinence, but they make the problem more bearable.

Behavioral treatment

Such nonmedical, nonsurgical methods consist of bladder training and exercise for the pelvic muscles. Bladder training is useful for urge and stress incontinence. Your doctor may have you drink more or less water and urinate according to a schedule in order to avoid problems. Exercises for the pelvic muscles, called Kegel exercises, help strengthen weakened muscles around the bladder. You'll be reminded always to squeeze your outlet muscle before standing up, bending, squatting, lifting, or doing anything else that causes leakage.

Behavioral techniques help reduce symptoms in up to 95 percent of properly chosen patients. Behavioral treatment is very useful because there are no side effects, and you can always proceed to another type of treatment.

Nutritional treatment

Food and drinks that can irritate the bladder are avoided. These include highly spiced foods, tomatoes, citrus fruits, chocolate, alcohol, milk, as well as cola drinks, coffee, tea, and other caffeinated beverages.

Biofeedback

In this treatment, you exert influence over parts of the body that you may not have realized you can control. Some doctors use a rectal balloon probe to produce wavy lines on paper, representing abdominal and sphincter pressures. Patients watch the printouts as they attempt to improve their sphincter contractions. Some studies have shown good, but limited, results.

Medical treatment

Medications are used to help eliminate infections that cause urinary problems, to stop abnormal contractions of the bladder muscles, and to tighten up weakened sphincter muscles. As many as 75 percent of properly chosen patients can be helped by these medications. Drugs used include propantheline bromide, flavoxate, phenylpropanolamine, and pseudoephedrine. Unfortunately, all medicines may have some side effects.

Electrical stimulation

No one knows exactly why, but applying an electrical current helps certain men to control mild to moderate stress incontinence.

Periurethral injections

Various substances, including Teflon, have been used throughout the years to "firm up" the urethra. (This is an old idea, dating back to the early 1960s.) Collagen injections are also used.

Surgical treatment

Portions of the prostate gland that may be pressing against the bladder or prostatic urethra can be cut away, and weak pelvic muscles can be reinforced or supported. There are many surgeries for incontinence, depending upon the cause of the problem. Surgeons can even implant artificial sphincters. Of course, all surgeries are risky because they involve cutting into the body, and once surgery has been performed, it cannot easily be undone, especially if something has been removed.

Healing through time

A final treatment is simply giving yourself time. In a fair number of men, urinary control will gradually reappear in the months following surgery as damaged nerves apparently repair themselves.

As you can see, there are many ways to deal with incontinence. Discuss all of the approaches with your doctor to see which is best for you. *If your doctor seems uninterested in your incontinence or brushes you off with a suggestion to wear pads, consider a new physician.*

Exercises to Improve Bladder Control

Kegel exercises have helped many men and women suffering from incontinence. The following information is quoted from a brochure called "Pelvic Muscle Exercises to Improve Your Bladder Control," prepared by HIP (Help for Incontinent People).[1]

Pelvic muscle exercises, also called Kegel (KAY-gull) exercises after Dr. Arnold Kegel who developed them, strengthen the pelvic floor muscles. These muscles contract and relax under your command to control the opening and closing of your bladder. When they are weak, urine leakage may result. However, through regular exercise, you can build up their strength and endurance and, in many cases, regain bladder control. Ask your doctor to discuss the following exercises with you.

Begin by Locating the Muscles to Be Exercised:

1. As you begin urinating, try to stop or slow the urine without tensing the muscles of your legs, buttocks, or abdomen. It is very important *not* to use these other muscles, because only the pelvic floor muscles help with bladder control.
2. When you are able to slow or stop the stream of urine, you have located the correct muscles. Feel the sensation of the muscles pulling inward and upward.

   Tip: Squeeze in the rectal area to tighten the anus, as if trying not to pass gas. You will be using the correct muscles.

Now You Are Ready to Perform the Exercise:

1. When you have located the correct muscles, set aside three to four times each day for exercising: morning, midday, and evening.
2. Squeeze your muscles to the slow count of four. Then, relax these muscles completely to the slow count of four. (Each four-second contraction and four-second relaxation makes one "set.")
3. Complete ten sets of these exercises during each of your daily exercise sessions.

(continued)

(Continued from previous page)

Here are some helpful tips:

- If your pelvic floor muscles are very weak, you should begin by contracting the muscles for only three to five seconds. Do the best you can and continue faithfully. In a few weeks, you should be able to increase the amount of time you are able to hold the contraction as well as the number of exercise sets you are able to do. Your goal is to hold each contraction for ten seconds, to relax for ten seconds, and to complete twenty-five to thirty sets.

- In the beginning, check yourself frequently by looking into the mirror and/or by placing a hand on your abdomen and buttocks to ensure that you do not feel your belly, thigh, or buttock muscles move. If there is movement, continue to experiment until you have isolated just the muscles of the pelvic floor.

- Your bladder control should begin to improve in three to four weeks. If you keep a record of urine leakage each day, you should soon notice fewer incidences.

Make Pelvic Muscle Exercises a Part of Your Daily Routine:

- Whether you are doing pelvic muscle exercises to improve or maintain bladder control, you must do them regularly on a life-time basis.

- Use daily routines such as watching TV, reading, stopping at traffic lights, and waiting in the grocery checkout line as cues to perform a few exercises.

Ten Healthy Habits to Help Improve Your Bladder Control:

1. Use the toilet regularly. Make toilet facilities convenient; this may mean a bedside commode, or a bedpan, or a urinal placed in the bed.
2. Wear clothes that are easy to remove when it is time to use the toilet.

(continued)

(Continued from previous page)

3. Train your bladder. Use a clock to schedule times to use the toilet. Plan to go every hour, then every 1½ hours, and so on, until you achieve a satisfactory schedule. Avoid frequent trips to the toilet "just in case."
4. Remain at the toilet until you feel your bladder is completely empty.
5. Empty your bladder before you start on a trip that will take an hour or more. Don't try to wait until you get home or until it's more convenient.
6. Learn to squeeze before you sneeze—and before you cough, laugh, get out of a chair, or pick up something heavy.
7. Establish regular bowel habits. Constipation affects bladder control.
8. Avoid foods that are known to affect the bladder, such as tomatoes, chocolate, spicy foods, alcohol, and beverages containing caffeine.
9. Watch your weight. Obesity makes bladder control more difficult. Ask your doctor about a sensible diet if you are overweight.
10. Stop smoking. Smoking is irritating to the bladder, and a smoker's cough may cause bladder leakage.

DEALING WITH ERECTILE DYSFUNCTION

Unfortunately, regardless of the treatment, a certain number of men will suffer from an inability to have an erection. Depending on the type of therapy used, as many as 50 to 60 percent of men will suffer from at least short-term impotence. For many, it will be permanent.

On the other hand, the word "permanent" no longer means forever. Here's a brief look at some helpful techniques.

Injections

The injection of a substance called PGE directly into the base of the penis, using a fine needle, produces satisfactory erections in most men.

It is important that both patient and doctor work closely together to find the exact dose that produces an erection. Patients tell me that, when PGE works well, they have a satisfactory erection for as long as forty-five minutes. In fact, many have told me that their erections actually last longer than they did before.

The initial injection is given by the doctor; after that, the patient self-injects himself at home, at the appropriate time.

One of the dangers with the injections is priapism, a condition in which the penis continues to remain hard for hours. It is important that the doctor tell the patient to seek medical help if the erection lasts for up to three to four hours, lest serious injury or gangrene of the penis occur.

PGE is mentioned here, but doctors use various substances for the injections.

All injections must be done carefully, under the guidance of a well-informed physician.

Vacuum Devices

The vacuum device has been around for years, dating back to the ads in *Police Gazette* magazine in the 1930s. The flaccid penis is put into a cylinder, and the air is pumped out of the cylinder, generally causing an erection. A constricting band is put around the base of the penis to trap the blood in the penis, keeping the penis hard. (This may not be the most appealing of techniques.)

Implants

For the past ten to twelve years, some surgeons have been using implants to help men with impotence. There are several different styles, but they work on the same basic principles.

The devices are like long, thin tubes, which are surgically implanted into the spongy part of the penis (on the underside, on each side of the urethral tube). There are two general types: one semirigid at all times, the other inflatable (like a life jacket).

Some complications resulting from the use of these devices include infections, narrowing of the urethra, and deformities of the penis. Further, many of the devices have had to be removed, often resulting in shrinkage of the penis.

DEALING WITH PAIN

Pain is often a side effect of cancer. Considering that approximately eight million Americans have contracted cancer, pain is a major problem, made worse by the fact that it is frequently undertreated in both adults and children.

Cancer can cause pain in several different ways, depending upon where it is located. If your cancer has spread beyond your prostate, it may be pressing on bones, organs, or nerves. Bone pain associated with cancer can be quite severe. Pain can result if the tumor blocks an organ or tube somewhere in the body, or if the cancer causes an infection or inflammation. Also, pain can occur if the cancer has slowed you down, and you've become stiff or weak. And some pain may be due to surgery or to the effects of radiation.

Pain is perhaps one of the most frightening aspects of cancer. Many patients say that they fear the pain they anticipate much more than they fear their cancer, or even dying. But as terrible as cancer pain sounds, a great deal of it can be effectively managed with modern medications, biofeedback, heat or cold packs, massage, nutrition, breathing and relaxation techniques, and other approaches—including surgery, nerve blocks, and even radiation.

Pain causes patients to suffer unnecessarily. It can:

- interfere with sleep, making one feel even more miserable
- upset the appetite, causing weight loss and malnutrition
- cause patients to cut back on their physical activities, which can hamper recovery, and
- contribute to depression and feelings of helplessness and hopelessness

Cancer pain must be recognized and treated.

Talk about Your Pain

Don't be afraid to tell the doctor that you hurt! Quiet patients who don't complain to their doctors are *not being good to themselves*. I worry about patients who never ask me about ways of dealing with pain, for "taking it like a man" can be very self-destructive. The best patient is the one who continually tells his doctor how he is feeling, because the doctor cannot treat a patient properly without knowing *everything* the patient is feeling, both physically and emotionally. The best patient communicates well, and demands the best from his doctors.

Medications for Pain

For mild pain

Aspirin, ibuprofen (such as Motrin), acetaminophen (Tylenol), and other nonprescription medicines are often helpful. You can purchase these medicines at a drugstore.

The side effects of aspirin include abdominal pain, gastritis, ulcers, and gastrointestinal bleeding. Use the coated aspirin that doesn't dissolve in the stomach or upper duodenum.

The side effects of ibuprofen include gastric ulceration, pain, and bleeding.

In recommended doses, acetaminophen (such as Tylenol) is usually well tolerated. However, an overdose can lead to the death of liver cells (hepatic necrosis). Kidney damage may occur with chronic overdosage, or with just chronic use in susceptible patients. Therefore, if you have kidney or liver abnormalities, take Tylenol with caution, or not at all. Be sure to discuss your Tylenol use with your doctor.

For moderate to severe pain

You may need prescription NSAIDs (nonsteroidal anti-inflammatory drugs) such as ketoprofen (Orudis) or fenoprofen calcium (Nalfon). NSAIDs can cause side effects such as bleeding and liver and kidney damage.

You may also need opioids such as morphine or codeine. These medicines, which require a prescription, are sometimes used in combination with the nonopioids mentioned above. The side effects of opioids include nausea, vomiting, constipation, mental "dulling," respiratory depression, dry mouth, urinary problems, sexual dysfunction, and sleepiness. You should not attempt to drive a car or operate machinery while taking opioids.

For swelling or pain related to swelling

Steroids—prescription medicines—such as prednisone may be used.

The side effects of steroids include the buildup of fluid in the body, bleeding, stomach irritation, interference with protein synthesis, and suppression of the immune system.

The various medicines may be given as pills, liquids, rectal suppositories (a pill placed in and absorbed by the rectum), shots (injections into the muscle), IV injections (through small needles inserted directly into a vein), epidural or intrathecal injections (injections into the back), or subcutaneous injections (a small needle placed directly under the skin).

Begin with the least powerful, least harmful, least invasive pain treatments possible, then move up to more powerful or invasive treatments if necessary.

Nonmedicine Treatments for Pain

Although they may sound simplistic, the nonmedicine treatments for pain can be very effective for many people. The nonmedicine treatments can be as simple as distracting yourself with good music, with conversation with good friends, or by watching television or videotapes. Your pain is still there but your mind is temporarily elsewhere, and the pain does not register. If it does register, if may be less intense.

Other nonmedicine treatments for pain include hot and cold packs, mild exercise or activity, massage, pressure, vibration, TENS (transcutaneous electrical nerve stimulation), biofeedback, acupuncture, hypnosis, imagery, and breathing and relaxation techniques. And rest is often a helpful remedy for many types of pain.

Psychotherapy or support groups are also helpful for many. Talking about your pain, your disease, your hopes, and your fears can help you feel better. Speaking with other men who have already experienced, or are currently experiencing, the same thing is also very helpful.

An almost entirely overlooked nonmedicine treatment for pain is education. In my many years of treating patients, I've found that honestly and completely telling patients that yes, it will hurt, but no, the pain will not be unbearable, and yes, they can have any medication or treatment they want, significantly reduces the need for medicine or treatment. Pain is often related to fear and anxiety. Telling people exactly what to expect—when and why—often helps to reduce their fear and anxiety, and thus reduces their pain. Knowing that your physician cares and is available for your physical and emotional needs can be a wonderful painkiller.

"Heavy-Duty" Treatments for Pain

When medicine and nonmedicine treatments have failed, some heavy-duty options are available. However, patients should approach these therapies with caution, because the therapies themselves can sometimes produce pain. They include:

Surgery—To remove tumors that are pressing on other parts of the body, especially on nerves.

Neurosurgery—To cut the nerves that are carrying the pain message to the brain.

Nerve blocks—To block pain signals by injecting medicine directly into a nerve or the spine.

Radiation—To shrink a tumor that is causing pain.

Assessing Your Pain

You alone know how much you hurt. Doctors can't measure pain the way we measure, say, the PSA level; we can only listen to your description and act accordingly. Therefore, patients can best help their doctors by "listening" carefully to their pain and by learning all about it so that they can best describe it.

Many people find it helpful to keep a Pain Diary. They then show the diary to their doctor, explaining exactly what hurt when, how much, and possibly why. There is no standard form for a Pain Diary, but patients should simply record this information for each pain:

- Date
- Time
- Where pain struck
- Type of pain
- How much it hurt (on a scale of 0 to 10, with 0 being no pain and 10 being unbearable pain)
- What you were doing when the pain struck
- What you did for the pain, if anything
- How you felt a little while later

The Pain Diary helps you and your doctor analyze your pain and plan the treatment.

Your doctor may also ask you to complete a Pain Inventory, or you may wish to do one yourself to assist in assessment of your own pain and attitudes toward pain. A typical Pain Inventory (short form) looks like this:[2]

Part I: What is your pain like?

1. Where is your pain?

   _____

   _____

2. Describe what it feels like (aching, throbbing, tingling, sharp, dull, hammerlike, shooting, stabbing, etc.):

   _____

   _____

3. Has the pain changed in any way?

   _____

   _____

4. Does anything make the pain better or worse (eating, moving, taking medicine, standing, sitting, being hot or cold, being touched, getting upset, thinking about your cancer, etc.)?

   _____

   _____

Part II: How much does it hurt?

5. Circle the number that describes the *worst* your pain felt in the past 24 hours.

   0   1   2   3   4   5   6   7   8   9   10
   No Pain   Worst Possible
                                              Pain Imaginable

6. Circle the number that describes your pain *at its least bothersome* in the past 24 hours.

   0   1   2   3   4   5   6   7   8   9   10
   No Pain   Worst Possible
                                              Pain Imaginable

7. Circle the number that describes the *average* level of your pain.

   0   1   2   3   4   5   6   7   8   9   10
   No Pain   Worst Possible
                                              Pain Imaginable

8. Circle the number that describes your pain *right now*.

   0   1   2   3   4   5   6   7   8   9   10
   No Pain   Worst Possible
                                              Pain Imaginable

9. Please make any comments you like about the intensity of your pain:

_____

_____

_____

_____

Part III: What does your pain do to you?

10. *General Activity:* In the past 24 hours, how much has your pain interfered with your general activity?

    0   1   2   3   4   5   6   7   8   9   10
    Not at All   Completely

11. *Normal Work:* In the past 24 hours, how much has your pain interfered with your normal work? This includes your work outside the home and your housework.

    0   1   2   3   4   5   6   7   8   9   10
    Not at All   Completely

12. *Ability to Walk:* In the past 24 hours, how much has your pain interfered with your ability to walk?

    0   1   2   3   4   5   6   7   8   9   10
    Not at All   Completely

13. *Mood:* In the past 24 hours, how much has your pain interfered with your mood?

    0   1   2   3   4   5   6   7   8   9   10
    Not at All   Completely

14. *Relations with Other People:* In the past 24 hours, how much has your pain interfered with your normal relations with other people?

    0   1   2   3   4   5   6   7   8   9   10
    Not at All   Completely

15. *Sleep:* In the past 24 hours, how much has your pain interfered with your regular sleep?

    0   1   2   3   4   5   6   7   8   9   10
    Not at All   Completely

16. *Ability to Enjoy Life:* In the past 24 hours, how much has your pain interfered with your normal enjoyment of life?

    0   1   2   3   4   5   6   7   8   9   10
    Not at All   Completely

17. *Sexual Relations:* In the past 24 hours, how much has your pain interfered with your normal sexual relations?

  0   1   2   3   4   5   6   7   8   9   10

Not at All   Completely

Part IV: Is your treatment helping?

18. What are your doctors doing for your pain (medications and treatments)?

_____

_____

_____

_____

_____

19. How much have the treatments or medicines your doctor has given you helped overall?

0% 10% 20% 30% 40% 50% 60% 70% 80% 90% 100%

No Relief   Complete

                                                 Relief

20. How much do your doctor's treatments help *immediately after* treatment (within a few hours of treatments)?

  0   1   2   3   4   5   6   7   8   9   10

Not at All   Completely

21. How much do your doctor's treatments help *a while after* treatment?

  0   1   2   3   4   5   6   7   8   9   10

Not at All   Completely

22. What are *you* doing for your pain (anything else you are taking, such as vitamins, herbs, or nonprescription medicines; anything else you are doing for your pain, such as exercising, soaking in a hot tub, etc.)?

_____

_____

_____

In my many years of treating patients, I have found that there is almost always a way to ameliorate the pain and emotional distress that accompany serious conditions. The keys to success are a constant flow of honest communication, a brave and caring physician, and a patient determined to triumph. Talking with other men in the same situation can also be very helpful, as we'll see in the next chapter.

10

Honest Talk from Men Who Have Been through It

E very man who must make a decision regarding his prostate cancer should talk to other men who have had the disease. Doctors and books can give you all kinds of information and statistics, but only a man who has been there can tell you what it's like to go under the knife, to be radiated, or to refuse treatment. Only a man whose nerve bundles have been damaged can tell you what it's like to temporarily or permanently lose the ability to have an erection.

Talking with my own patients, and listening to men as they open up at prostate support groups, has always been an educational experience. Some of their stories are sad, some are humorous. Some are frightening, and a few are inspirational. Let's listen in on some of the men who have been treated, some who have refused treatment, and others who have not yet decided what to do.

GETTING THE NEWS—AND WHAT TO DO NEXT

"I was devastated," said one man, a seventy-two-year-old teacher who was told that he had cancer seven years ago.

"It felt like my life was over. I literally cried," confessed Lou, who was sixty-five when he got the news. "I actually got the news the day I retired. The kids were grown up, the house was paid off, and I had a nice pension. I was looking forward to living the life of Riley, and wham! I got cancer."

Dan, a forty-five-year-old construction worker, said: "I knew I had it. My dad and brother had it. I guess I was ready for the diagnosis. I mean, well, you *know*."

Senate Majority Leader Robert Dole learned that he had prostate cancer following a routine physical examination. The only symptom he had was nocturia (getting up to urinate often at night). "I'm a fairly strong person," he said, "but you're sort of stunned. . . . I was just overwhelmed."[1]

Learning that he has cancer feels like a kick in the gut to almost every man. But what he does once he gets the news is important. Most men go along with their doctors' recommendations, literally placing their lives in the hands of strangers. For a while, a man may feel that he has lost control of his life as he submits to rounds of tests and consultations, then to the treatment and its aftermath.

Other men prefer to look upon their cancer as a challenge. Determined to stay in control of their lives, they insist upon choosing their own treatments.

Still others look upon the news as a call to arms. "It's a war," said fifty-nine-year-old Stan. "It's me against the bleeping cancer. Only one of us is going to win, and it's going to be me!" When asked how he intended to wage the war, Stan replied: "Learn everything there is to learn."

Is one attitude better than another? I think so. In almost forty years of treating patients, I've found that those who decide to fight the disease, those who want to maintain control over their lives, and those who look upon the disease as a challenge tend to do better than those who meekly surrender. In fact, it's the patients who give their doctors the most trouble, the ones who challenge treatment choices, who ask the most questions, and who refuse to play helpless that do the best.

One other type of patient also tends to do well: the older man who has lived a full, satisfying life, and who accepts the fact that his time upon this earth is coming to a close. Declining strong measures, he puts his affairs in order and gracefully accepts. His last days or months are usually filled with touching good-byes and tributes to and from his family and friends.

SATISFIED AND UNHAPPY PATIENTS

Men's physical responses to and opinions of their treatments vary. Some are pleased, while others are dissatisfied, even angry. Even when the therapy goes well, some men are unhappy, while others take their troubles in stride. General Norman Schwarzkopf, of Desert Storm fame, underwent a nerve-sparing prostatectomy in May 1994. Seven months later, the sixty-year-old said that he feels "like a million dollars. . . . Everything is absolutely, totally back to normal."[2]

Some men are satisfied despite less than optimal results of treatment. Jerry is a very pleasant-looking sixty-three-year-old engineer whose wife developed lung cancer just before he found out that he had prostate cancer. Despite this double disaster, Jerry remains positive about his future. He sailed through surgery and is looking forward to trying out injections to restore his potency. Here's what he told me (my questions are in bold italics):

> *I'll start back in 1990. I went to the doctor, and he determined that my prostate was, oh, five times as big as it should be. The only symptom I had was that when I went to urinate, it was very bloody. The doctor decided to do a PSA and a biopsy. It was all negative. After that, I had a PSA every six months, and I had a total of three biopsies—all negative. But my PSA was slowly creeping up from 8 to 9.*
>
> *Finally, in 1994, the doctor said, "Let's do another biopsy. And this time I'm going to do four on each side." Sure enough, they came back positive. He said the cancer might have been there before, but I don't see how he could have missed it with the previous three biopsies.*
>
> *The way my doctor explained it to me, there's only one cure for prostate cancer. If it hasn't escaped from the prostate, take it out. I had the surgery a month ago, and I've only had the catheter out for two weeks. My control is already coming back, especially at night. I've been working on my exercises.*
>
> ***How about the sexual complications?*** *We sat down and talked about it, and the doctor explained the different methods I could try after surgery. When I'm ready, I'm going to try the injection method. I don't see why the impotence won't improve as quickly as the incontinence did.*
>
> ***Knowing what you now know, would you go back and change your treatment if you could?*** *No. I would have done the same thing, even if the cancer had spread.*
>
> ***Do you have any advice for a man who has just learned that he has prostate cancer?*** *You've got to have a positive mental attitude. As soon as they let me know I had prostate cancer, I went to a support group. And I immediately started doing*

visualizations on killing the cancer cells, keeping them contained in the prostate.

Jerry was pleased and positive, but a fifty-seven-year-old business-man named Alvin is not at all happy with his treatment. Although his surgery was successful in that it apparently removed all of the cancerous cells, and his PSA remains low, Alvin is severely depressed by the surgery's side effects. He also feels that the doctors railroaded him into the operation.

I didn't have any symptoms, but at a regular checkup the doctor found that there was something wrong when he did the finger/rectal examination. My PSA was 38. The urologist told me that I had to have a biopsy, and when I did, he told me that I had to have surgery.

Did the doctor explain all of the options to you? *Yes, he did. But the way he explained the options, there* were *no options.*

Do you feel that the doctor's explanation was slanted in favor of surgery? *Yes. The doctor didn't explain nearly enough for me to fully understand what was going to happen.*

Are you sorry that you had the surgery? *I regret having the surgery. It turned my life upside down.*

Why is that? *They cut the nerve to my penis when they cut out my prostate. Physically, I can't have sexual relations because I can't have an erection. I have to give myself an injection to do anything.*

I also have a problem with leaking. If I sneeze or cough, I leak. If I try to lift something, my pants get wet. It's depressing; it's embarrassing.

It is all psychologically very painful. With the urine problem and the sex problem, I'm depressed to the point that I just don't want to stay alive anymore. I wish they had just cut off my penis and testicles; then I would be done with it entirely.

IS A RADICAL PROSTATECTOMY WORTH HAVING?

The number of radical prostatectomies has been increasing rapidly in the past few years. Despite the controversy as to which men will benefit from the surgery, the stage at which the cancer should be surgically removed, and even whether surgery is better than doing nothing at all, growing numbers of men are sacrificing their prostates. I've already discussed the potential benefits and risks, but there's nothing like hearing from men who have been under the surgeon's knife. Sixty-three-year-old Thomas came through his surgery with ease:

Well, my cancer was found back in early '91. I had some problems peeing, so the doctor stuck his finger up my whatsit and said I had the "big C." So I had the surgery, the one where they cut out the whole prostate. It went like clockwork. I hardly had any pain, I was up and around real soon, and I went home in three days. I could pee in a couple weeks. I couldn't use my thingie with my wife after the surgery, but that was OK.

You didn't mind losing your ability to have an erection? *It was either that or die. Anyway, I had another surgery to put in a pumplike thing, so now I'm working fine. Just pump it up, and it works fine.*

You know, I interviewed four doctors before letting one cut me open. I got the best mechanic for my car, the best accountant for my taxes, and the best doc to cut me open. The other thing is my attitude. Some men bellyache and moan about everything, and that makes them hurt more. Me, I think about how good it's going to be.

I wish everyone could be as satisfied with his surgery as Thomas was. Unfortunately, some men, like Frank, are angry with their surgeons:

God, if I could get that son of a bitch alone, I'd fix it so he needs *surgery!*

Why are you so upset? *Because that lousy bastard led me to believe that everything would be fine, but it wasn't. I think he was lying to me. He spouted all these statistics about how great the surgery would be. He said the risks were minimal. Well, now I'm a "minimal" guy. I've got minimal control over my urine, I can only get a minimal erection, and I've got a minimal chance of living, because the surgery didn't work. My PSA is coming back up. He botched the surgery. Either that or the cancer had already moved out of the prostate before the surgery, in which case the bastard botched the diagnosis. I called some attorneys. I'm gonna nail his hide to the wall!*

If you could go back in time, what would you want your doctor to do differently? I'd want him to tell me the truth! If it's going to be bad news, I can learn to live with it. But don't tell me it's going to be wonderful. Damn! Don't lie to me!

DOCTOR–PATIENT COMMUNICATION IS IMPORTANT

Frank very angrily expresses what a good number of men feel to a lesser degree: that their doctors either sugarcoat the truth in their discussions, steer their patients toward only one treatment, or simply don't listen to their patients enough.

Fifty-two-year-old Sam keeps telling the story of his encounter with an arrogant, uncommunicative urologist:

I was diagnosed in 1988, when I went to the doctor because of urinary problems. My internist sent me to a urologist. "You're seeing the best urologist around," my doctor told me.

So I went to the urologist. When I asked him what my PSA was, he ignored me, and went right on talking. So I asked him again, and he ignored me. Then I said, "Look, Doc, I asked you a question. What's my PSA?" You know what he said? He said, "You don't need to know that."

When I said that I did need to know it, he dropped my file on the floor and walked out of the room! He just walked right out of the room! I couldn't believe it! Like I'm a piece of dirt, that's how he treated me.

Forty-nine-year-old Paul, an attorney, also had problems with uncommunicative doctors. Although tempted to sue at first, he decided instead to make it *his job* to get his doctors to communicate properly.

I found it best to study up as much as possible before speaking to my doctors, and to prepare lists of questions. This demonstrated my seriousness. It also showed them that I appreciated the fact that time is money, and that I was willing to focus the conversation as much as possible. I also made it very clear to the doctors—very respectfully—that it was their job to answer all of my questions. I always sat up tall in my chair. I looked the doctor right in the eye when we spoke. I spoke firmly and clearly. I rephrased what they said to show them that I was listening, and that I understood. If the telephone rang when we were speaking, I told them that I would appreciate it if they would focus on me, for I was in their office at the scheduled time. If they ever stood up to signal that the interview was over, I remained sitting, notebook in hand, and asked the next question.

This approach worked with most of the doctors. When they see that you will not be denied, they usually back down and speak to you. The key is to erase the cultural perception that doctors are godlike creatures to whom we must be terribly subservient. Treat them like you would a tutor you hire to teach you French. You would demand the best from the tutor, wouldn't you? Demand the best from your doctor. After all, you're the one who's paying.

IS THERE SEX AFTER A RADICAL PROSTATECTOMY?

Most men being treated or counseled have said that one of their great fears before surgery was that they would lose the ability to have an erection. "I won't be a man anymore," some said, or "What will I do when I can't do it?"

The cold, hard statistics are not encouraging: A good number of men will partially or completely lose the ability to have a satisfactory erection. Some men regain their prowess with the passing of several months; others never do. Fifty-two-year-old Zach, a banker from New York, speaks for many men when he says:

I just don't feel like much of a man anymore. Yeah, I know it's all a bunch of male chauvinistic, testosterone-driven, macho crap, but the truth is I don't feel like much of a man anymore. A man is certainly not defined by his erection, and he may not even use it much, but I sure miss it now that it's gone. If I had to do it over again, I'd take my chances with the cancer.

Fifty-seven-year-old Ken talks about his experiences with sex following his radical prostatectomy. He's found that using an injection to make his penis erect is a workable substitute for a fully functioning penis:

Since I'm not taking hormonal drugs at this time, I still have a libido. I still get partial erections, and I augment them with a drug called prostaglandin. It works wonders for me.

Of course, sex is not as spontaneous as it used to be. But when you get to be my age—I'll be fifty-eight in a couple months—it's more preplanned anyway. So that doesn't seem to be a problem.

Howard, a strong and friendly sixty-two-year-old grocery store manager, had a prosthetic device implanted six months after his radical prostatectomy. He's delighted with the results:

I'll tell you this, impotence makes you feel bad. Your thing just goes to nothing. Then you get this implant; it really gives you a new lease on life. You have to remember that sex was pretty unsatisfactory for three or four years prior to the surgery. Then I became the bionic man, a real tiger! Here, at sixty-two, I'm like a nineteen-year-old guy. I can go all night! It's been about a year and a half since I had the implant. I really recommend it to any man.

The only thing is, you lose some of your size. And it takes a while for you to get used to your pants rubbing up against it. Now, I'm getting used to it so I'm simmering down, which my wife thinks is a godsend. The doctor tells me that some guys don't experience ejaculation at all. In my case I do, but it's a long time in coming. But it's great. I'm a tiger.

A small number of men who are able to have a nerve-sparing radical prostatectomy still manage to come through the surgery with the vital nerves intact, or only partially damaged. Here's how Peter and Kate have described their experience:[3]

Even though the urologist said there was a good chance the cancerous lump could be successfully removed by surgery, we knew that such an operation "down there" might seriously hamper, if not end, our flourishing love life.

The surgeon said he would try to peel the cancerous prostate gland off the nerve bundle underneath, which is vital to a man's being able to have an erection.

The operation was successful. We were told that it would take time, anywhere from several months to more than a year, before we could expect workable erections. Even then, the erection process could be "iffy" because of Peter's age [then sixty-two, now sixty-seven].

Performance anxiety, as every man knows, can feed on itself and begin to eat away at the other elements that bind a couple together. . . .

By talking to each other, we found that there are all sorts of loving, exciting things we could do to express ourselves sexually and emotionally. It is vitally important not to become isolated from each other by pretending it doesn't matter and by making excuses to avoid the loaded "performance" problem.

We lightened up, had fun in bed, experimented with massage, new positions, new techniques. When an erection wasn't forthcoming, each of us could still have an orgasm.

In time, workable erections came back. Are they as frequent and as dependable as before the operation? Not quite. But in many ways our lovemaking is even better than before because we have an expanded romantic repertoire that includes such things as frequent, lingering hugs and kisses and all sorts of imaginative things enamored couples can do behind closed doors.

The key: Learn to relax and keep talking to each other openly, clearly, honestly, and lovingly.

Forty-nine-year-old Lewis has this very practical advice for men who are afraid of becoming impotent:

I would ask them to consider the alternative. A wife's main concern is to have her husband alive, not to visit him in the cemetery.

WHAT HAPPENS WHEN TREATMENTS DON'T WORK?

Jack is a gentle, soft-spoken man with a full head of thick black hair. Both a radical prostatectomy and radiation treatment failed to cure his cancer. Now he's on hormone therapy, and his PSA is stable. Jack wishes his doctors had better prepared him for the possibility of side effects by explaining everything to him.

I was diagnosed as having prostate cancer in August of 1990, and had the surgery in December 1990. After sixteen months, my PSA level started to rise again, so my urologist sent me to an oncologist, who recommended radiotherapy. I had the radioactive treatments for seven weeks, five days a week. When I started, my PSA level was eight and a half, and when I ended seven weeks later, it was still eight and a half. It just didn't do me any good.

A month after that I started on hormones. The hormone shots give me the sweats. I get those at any time of the day or night, and it's not a nice feeling. But, after the first month, my PSA was down to zero. And, I'm happy to tell you, it's been that way ever since.

Did the doctors tell you why the radiation didn't work? No.

They just said, "Sorry, it didn't work, so move on to a new treatment"? *Basically, that is correct. My foot, my ankle, and my calf are now swollen. That's directly from the radiation, they think.*

How do you feel about the treatment you received? *The only thing I would say that I am disturbed about is this: Any of the questions that you would ask any of the doctors, they would, of course, answer. However, there are many questions that you might not know enough to ask. And doctors don't volunteer much information. I don't know if it would have made any difference in my thinking, but I would like to have known more. The doctor told me he would get all the cancer out, and it would be fine and dandy. Unfortunately, it was not that way.*

Seventy-one-year-old Howard reacted very calmly to the news that he still had cancer, despite surgery, radiation, and hormones.

I don't blame the doctors or the treatments or the "system." We're granted a finite amount of time on this earth, and when that time is up, it's up. I'm going to enjoy the time that I have left. I'd also like to make a contribution to the world before I go. I could help out at the retirement home as a way of saying "thank you" to the world before I go.

I met Ken at a prostate cancer support group meeting. A cheerful, energetic, and intelligent man, he suffered the double disappointment of finding first that he had prostate cancer and then that the radical prostatectomy did not remove all of the cancer. Follow-up radiation left him with urinary and sexual difficulties, as well as an unusual discharge from his rectum. He now feels that doctors rush patients into making their decision and don't tell them about all the alternatives. If he had to do it over again, Ken thinks that he would have radiation before surgery, hoping to shrink the tumor, thus making it possible for the doctors to remove the entire cancerous growth.

If I had to do it over again, I would do a couple of things differently. I believe that the only way to cure cancer is to take it out. If you can remove the infected cells, it's a cure. In most cases, that does not happen, even in "successful" surgeries like mine. That's why I would have undergone hormonal therapy first, either Lupron or Zoladex, for a period of three or four months prior to the surgery to shrink the prostate and the cancer. Then remove the prostate and the entire cancer.

They also gave me a transfusion after the surgery with my own infected blood. It was my blood, but it had some of my cancer cells in it. Most doctors say it's such a small volume of blood put back in that it doesn't matter, but I wouldn't chance it if I did it again. I'd use the common blood supply.

What would you say to a man who has just been told that he has prostate cancer? *I would advise him to do four things:*

One, do not succumb to pressure from the medical community to do something immediately.

Two, find the nearest prostate cancer support group and go for a couple of sessions. We're the people who have the problem; we're the people who have done the research. We probably know more about this than the doctors do. I would recommend that before anyone let a doctor cut him, zap him with radiation, or even give him hormones, he go to a group and listen to the men who have been there.

Three, try to downstage the cancer before surgery.

Four, do not use your own blood for a transfusion.

WHO SHOULD TRY ALTERNATIVE TREATMENTS?

Max is a lanky, intelligent man who believes that the medical system is overlooking viable treatments for prostate cancer. He thinks that doctors tend to "push" the treatments that they know and do, turning a blind eye to other approaches, whether standard or alternative. If he had to do it again, he would opt for alternative treatments. Here's what he says:

> There is evidence that the immune system can make a difference in cancer treatment, but who ever heard of combining immune therapy with other treatment modalities? There is strong anecdotal evidence that alternative treatments, such as Essiac tea, help. It is low-cost and has no side effects, so why not add it to the arsenal?
>
> **If you had to do it all over again, what would you do?** Knowing what I know today, I probably would not have a radical prostatectomy. I would use a combination of hormone therapy, hyperthermia, vitamins and minerals, and other substances. I've got the plan all mapped out. And when my PSA becomes elevated, I plan to follow it.

Dick, the satisfied patient whose story we've already read, is also interested in alternative treatment, but only as an adjunct to his primary treatment (radical prostatectomy). He explains:

> My wife got lung cancer when I got the prostate cancer. What are the odds of two people in the same household getting cancer at the same time? We come from two different genetic backgrounds, so there must be something else at work. So we've started changing our lifestyle. We are using visualization, meditation, and hypnosis, and are changing to a vegetarian diet. I also take a high dosage of vitamins C, 2,000 mg, and E, 400 IU, as well as a multimineral.

THE PSYCHOLOGY OF CANCER

In talking about the psychology of cancer, psychologist Kathleen Cairns, Psy.D., of Beverly Hills told me that men who just learned that they have cancer go through the same five stages experienced by people who learn they are going to die: denial, depression, anger, bargaining, and acceptance.

The news that one has cancer comes as an apparently irreversible, horrible truth. It is so beyond the realm of normal existence that we don't want to "let it into our minds"—we can't. Cancer is something that happens to other people, we tell ourselves, not to us.

Some men, such as Harvey, refuse to internalize the fact that they have cancer. Harvey is a broad-shouldered, rugged-looking sixty-nine-year-old former lumberjack who was reluctant to undergo testing because it might lead to bad news. He describes how he found out that he had prostate cancer:

My internist said I should see a urologist because of my symptoms. He told me it could be nothing or it could be serious, so I should get checked. So I thought yeah, yeah, sure, I'll get around to it. Six months later I went back to my internist because I was still having leakage after I went to the bathroom, and I couldn't keep it up well. And so he said, "Did you see the urologist?" I said, "No." I didn't make the appointment because I wasn't having any problems that I was really concerned with. And I was busy. Besides, I thought he was making a big deal out of a little problem. So I have to shake it twice, what's the big deal? A little more exercise, a few more oysters, and it will be all right.

Other men will study the situation with great determination, speaking to many doctors, reading everything they can, amassing a great store of knowledge in an attempt to gain control over their lives. These men are also in denial: not of their cancer, but of their emotions.

Most men go numb when they get the news. It hits them a few hours, a few days, a few weeks later. Reality seeps in and they are overwhelmed with depression and fear. There are many fears: fear of death, of not recovering, of not having the same life, of pain, of the unknown, of the treatment, of disfiguration, of loss of manhood, of loss of their wives. Some men go rapidly into a depression. They may become dependent, feeling very helpless. Often, they'll agree to whatever their doctor may suggest.

Sixty-five-year-old Albert, who had owned and run a small grocery story for thirty years, immediately agreed to the therapy that his doctor suggested. He still seems to be in shock: "When the doctor told me I had it, I was . . . I didn't know what to do. He told me about the surgery, and three days later he took it out. I don't even remember what I did in the three days."

As a physician, I've seen many men in the anger stage, although I tend to see them after they've been treated for their cancer. Then, their anger is usually directed at the doctor who they feel did a poor job, or who they feel recommended the wrong treatment. But I've seen only a few men in the bargaining stage. One was fifty-six-year-old Stan, who kept asking questions such as: "If I start jogging five miles a day, will that make it go away?" "If I give up meat, will it go away?" "What if I become a vegetarian and start exercising, what will that do?" These are all good questions, but considering that he had never before been interested in good health habits, they suggest that he was looking for a way out.

Dr. Cairns says that it is very normal for men to go through the five stages. It's just as normal for them to break the pattern by jumping ahead or moving back a stage or two. It's also very normal for men to linger in one stage or another before moving on.

The best thing a man can do, according to Dr. Cairns, is to allow himself to feel his feelings, to recognize that these are stages that he must move through and that he should stay in each stage as long as is natural for him. He shouldn't try to force himself to the fifth stage, acceptance. Instead, he should allow himself to arrive at acceptance when it is right for him to do so. And, always, he should surround himself with people who love and support him.

11

The Healthy Prostate Program, Part I: Prevention

There was a strong, healthy grandmother seventy-two years young who lived an active life, driving her friends to club meetings and to the store, working part-time and running errands for her sickly neighbors. One day she told me she had had a cold for three weeks; it simply wouldn't go away. When it persisted, I insisted she be thoroughly checked out. The diagnosis was grim: leukemia, a cancer of the white blood cells.

I visited her in the hospital every day, horrified at the rapid progress of the cancer. This once-vibrant woman lay in bed, too weak to move, mouth agape, eyes dull. Shortly before she died, she said to me, "I was so healthy. Why did I get sick?" Unable to answer her question, I turned away, tears in my eyes. I had no answers for her; neither could I offer her any help. It was especially painful because this woman was my mother.

Perhaps saddest of all is the fact that most cancers are preventable. The National Cancer Institute, the American Cancer Society, and other mainline organizations heartily agree with what I've been saying since the early 1970s: Prevention is the cure for most cancers. If we eat a good diet, if we don't smoke, and if we cut down on our exposure to hazardous substances, we can almost completely eliminate cancer. What's true for cancer is true for many, many other diseases. They are largely preventable. Yes, we will all sicken and pass away at some point, but most of us can live healthy and strong to a very old age, if we make prevention a regular part of our lives.

Many men ask me what they can do once they have a prostate problem. Fewer ask me what they can do to prevent problems from

187

occurring in the first place, which is too bad because prevention is always the best policy. There are steps we can take to reduce our risk of getting prostate cancer, infections, and prostatitis. Because we don't know exactly what causes benign prostatic hypertrophy (BPH), however, there are no specific preventive steps to take, just the same good health habits that keep your immune system—your "doctor within"—as strong as possible. I've put together a four-step Healthy Prostate Program for preventing prostate disease to help point my patients in the direction of good health. The steps are:

1. Be self-aware.
2. Have regular checkups.
3. Use your sexual smarts.
4. Keep your "doctor within" strong.

Although there is no guaranteed way to prevent all prostate problems, this four-step program can help reduce some of the risks by making you more likely to notice problems in the early stage, lowering your exposure to certain diseases, strengthening your immune system, and getting you to your physician for early treatment.

STEP ONE: BE SELF-AWARE

Prevention begins with awareness. Be aware of changes in your urinary or sexual habits, and understand that these changes may be symptoms of other problems. But don't worry *excessively* about minor, or even major, changes in your urinary or sexual habits, and don't jump to the conclusion that you have a dread disease. Just pay attention to your body and its habits, and have changes checked out by your doctor.

You should also be aware of the fact that other diseases may put you at risk for prostate problems. Having had gonorrhea, chlamydia, any other sexually transmitted disease (STD), any discharge from your penis, or kidney disease does not necessarily mean that you have or will have a prostate problem. But you should be aware of the fact that these diseases *may* lead to prostate problems, and you should make sure your doctor knows your full medical history.

STEP TWO: HAVE REGULAR CHECKUPS

For many years, as I taught physical diagnosis to medical students, I emphasized the importance of the digital rectal examination (DRE) in checking the prostate. Although the DRE has been challenged by the PSA and ultrasound, I still believe that the DRE should be a part of *every* complete physical examination performed on every adult male. It should be as routine as listening to a patient's heart.

Your doctor should do a baseline PSA when you hit forty to establish a reference point for future comparison. The PSA should be repeated immediately if any prostate abnormalities are found, or if any symptoms develop between the ages of forty and fifty. If the DRE or PSA is abnormal, a transrectal ultrasound should be performed.

Beginning at age fifty, men should have both the DRE and PSA performed yearly. (This should not be treated any differently than the Pap smear for women.) If either the DRE or PSA is abnormal, trans-rectal ultrasound should be performed immediately.

Along with these tests, which are specifically designed to pick up prostate problems, your doctor should perform a thorough examination, looking for any signs of immune-system weakness or other problems that might suggest an increased susceptibility to disease.

STEP THREE: USE YOUR SEXUAL SMARTS

Many years ago, when I was a buck private in the U.S. Army stationed in Italy, young soldiers only had to worry about getting syphilis and gonorrhea. Those were the only two sexually transmitted diseases (STDs) that concerned us back then (mostly because if you got caught with an STD, the army would throw you into the stockade!). Today, I wish we had only syphilis and gonorrhea to worry about. Now we must also be concerned about AIDS, herpes, chlamydia, genital candidiasis, genital warts, and other STDs. There are over twenty STDs, producing problems ranging from the very mild to the deadly. And because the prostate is part of a man's sexual apparatus, some STDs threaten that gland as well.

Abstinence is the best protection against all STDs. The next-best protection is a long-term, monogamous relationship with an equally monogamous partner. Here are some other tips for avoiding STDs:

- Use a latex condom, spermicides containing nonoxynol-9, or similar "protection." Contraceptive pills, diaphragms, and other contraceptive devices do not protect against STDs.
- Make sure you know your partner's sexual history. Every time you sleep with a person, you risk exposure to all the diseases that previous partners may have had.

- Be aware. Does your partner have genital or anal warts, sores, or other problems? Learn to recognize the signs of STDs.
- Check yourself regularly for discharges, sores, blisters, or rashes in the genital or anal areas. Be aware of any pain or discomfort in those or nearby areas. Be suspicious of any "flu" that seems to come out of nowhere, or that lasts too long. When in doubt, have yourself checked out by a doctor.
- Remember that the absence of any obvious symptoms does not prove that you are completely healthy. Have regular checkups even when you think you are in tip-top shape, just to be sure.

STEP FOUR: KEEP YOUR "DOCTOR WITHIN" STRONG

The great humanitarian, Nobel Prize laureate, and physician Albert Schweitzer once told a group of M.D.'s: "All of us have a doctor within. The patients come to us not knowing that truth. We are at our best when we help that doctor within."

Although no one can fully describe, define, or locate the doctor within, we do know that the immune system plays a major role. We also know that positive thinking, good nutrition, and exercise are excellent ways of boosting our immune systems.

#1: Strengthening the Doctor Within via the Mind-Body Connection

I once overheard an interesting conversation between two students at the UCLA Biomedical Library. One was tall and slim, the other rounded and short. The tall man said to his friend: "I'm a psychology major, and I know that the body is the body and the mind is the mind. There's no mind-body connection!"

"Think about this," the shorter man replied. "Imagine that you're at the library late tonight. This gorgeous girl sits down next to you. She has long dark hair, an open blouse with lots of cleavage. She smiles at you, a big smile. You start talking, and a few minutes later you go way to the back of the library. It's just you and her. She unbuttons her blouse and she's not wearing a bra."

The shorter man interrupted his steamy story to ask his tall friend: "Do you have an erection right now?" The tall student nodded, embarrassed.

"Has any girl undressed in front of you, or touched you?" The tall man shook his head.

"Then tell me," challenged the short fellow. "What, besides your thoughts, gave you that erection? Nothing. It was all in your mind."

There is no doubt that the human mind and body are intimately connected, and that we can use the connection either to our advantage or to our detriment. In fact, we already do use it, if unknowingly. There is a very easy way to strengthen the immune system and the body: self-administering our "mental medication."

Your daily R$_x$

Your daily mental medicine prescription is very simple: Think good thoughts and avoid unhappy ones. If you're not in the habit of thinking good thoughts, make a conscious effort to take your "mental medicine" three times a day by saying, out loud, something nice, happy, pleasant, loving, supportive, or positive.

If you're not sure what to say, you can use or modify some of the affirmations below. Affirmations are brief, positive statements painting verbal pictures of the events or things you want to occur. They steer your thoughts in the right direction by asserting only the positive. Affirmations put you on the road to success by planting positive seeds in your mind. Since every thought that enters your mind is acted upon, the more affirmations you recite, the better. Here are some samples:

Today's a great day, filled with opportunities for happiness and success.

I'm permitting only positive thoughts to form in my mind, thoughts of love, happiness, and health. . . .

I am filled with love, love of life and love of others. . . .

"Mental medicine" is nontoxic, has no side effects, and tends to grow stronger with each dosage.

To help you take your mental medicine . . .

Sometimes it's difficult to remain calm and to keep the negative out of our minds. Here are Nine Tips for Keeping the Negatives Out:

1. *Turn confrontations into consultations*—If someone wants to tell you what a jerk you are, pay attention. Don't get mad, don't fight back, actually listen. If you don't learn something about yourself, you will at

least defuse the situation by appearing to be interested in what he or she has to say.

2. *Turn bad situations to good*—With a little thought, you can often find a way to make the most out of an unpleasant situation. For example, carry your favorite music tapes or books on tape in your car. If you're caught in traffic, pop the tapes into the cassette player. Instead of stewing over the traffic, you can listen to some great music or "read" an exciting book.

3. *Turn failure into a challenge*—One of my sons was the absolute worst baseball player in the neighborhood when he was a little boy. I remember watching, filled with pain, as the other boys laughed at him each time he struck out or dropped a ball (which was often). Rather than give up, Barry decided to become the best ballplayer around. He spent one entire winter hitting little rocks with a baseball bat and throwing a rubber ball against the garage door. By the time spring rolled around, he had become skilled, and he was later the Most Valuable Player on his Little League and a member of the All-Star team. He turned failure into success by viewing failure as a challenge.

4. *Turn difficulties into an opportunity for self-assessment*—If you keep getting fired from your jobs, ask yourself why rather than rail against the "unfair system" and "those lousy bosses." Perhaps you're in the wrong line of business, perhaps you don't have the necessary skills or education, perhaps you have a bad attitude toward work. Or maybe you're just not cut out to work for others; maybe you should be your own boss. And if you've been divorced four times, isn't it time to ask yourself what you may be doing wrong, instead of simply assuming that all women or men are rotten?

5. *Don't let lack of opportunity hold you back*—Many people have told me that they would have been a doctor/attorney/athlete/scientist/businessperson, but their parents didn't have enough money to send them to school, or didn't introduce them to the right people. But lack of anything need not hold anyone back. Remember that Abraham Lincoln was born in a log cabin, and Olympic hero Jesse Owens, from a sharecropper family, began picking cotton in the fields at the age of seven.

6. *Prevent disasters by planning fallbacks*—Not too long ago I met a young man who wants to be a playwright. He told me that "supporting oneself as a playwright is next to impossible, so I took journalism classes while studying theater in college. Now I work as a reporter, earning a decent living while I work on my plays at night. If I make it as a playwright, great. If not, at least I'm doing my second-favorite kind of writing."

7. *Know that difficulties, setbacks, and outright failures are a normal part of life, even for the most successful of us*—President Harry Truman was a failed businessman before becoming Vice President of the United States, and was written off by practically everyone in the 1948 presidential election (which he won). Babe Ruth, the great home run hitter, was also the strikeout king of baseball. Thomas Edison failed hundreds of times before finding the right filament for his lightbulb. Failure is a part of everyone's life. For many of us, failure is the first step on the road to success. Or, as Henry Ford has said: "Failure is the opportunity to begin again more intelligently."

8. *Keep your eye firmly on your goals*—Don't let adversity or setbacks stop you.

9. *Finally, never give in*—A very wise man once said that a winner is like a boxer who keeps getting knocked down, but is too dumb to know that he's lost. A few people succeed instantly because of talent, luck, opportunity, or whatever. The rest of the world's greats won because they didn't know they were losing. They simply set their eyes on their goals, and never gave up.

#2: Feeding Your Doctor Within

Generous doses of "mind medicine" aren't the only way we can strengthen our doctor within. We can also give the doctor the best raw materials possible to work with while striving to keep our bodies in good running order. Those raw materials are, of course, the foods we eat.

Nutrition plays an important role in health. One of the first nutritional studies was recorded thousands of years ago in the biblical book of Daniel 1:5–16. Daniel and other young men had been brought to the court of King Nebuchadnezzar of Babylon, where they were to be educated and raised. Nebuchadnezzar ordered that the youths be fed the same rich foods that he ate. But Daniel asked the king's steward if he and his three friends could eat only vegetables, grains, and water. At first the steward refused, fearing that if Daniel and his friends ate these "lesser" foods, they would become ill, and his head would roll. But Daniel proposed an experiment: He and his friends would eat only vegetables, grains, and water for ten days, then be compared to the other youths, who would enjoy the king's food. At the end of the ten-day trial period, it was agreed that Daniel and his friends actually looked healthier than the others, so they were allowed to continue eating their poor man's diet.

Daniel may not have known about cholesterol, vitamins, glucose, and other nutritional components of food. Nor was it likely that he was aware of the effects of excessive dietary fat, sugar, and other components of food on the immune system and the body. He just knew that "poor" food was actually more healthful than the "rich" food most people craved. We still crave rich foods today. Here in the United States we eat the Standard American Diet (SAD), the modern equivalent of the king's diet. Full of excess calories, fat, cholesterol, sugar, and other items, the SAD taxes our immune systems and bodies. The globs of fat we eat are especially encouraging to cancer. Those of us eating the SAD get 45 percent or more of our calories from fat. Only 35 percent of our calories come from carbohydrates, but most of these are refined carbohydrates (sugar). Seventy-five percent of typical SAD foods are processed, and the SAD averages some 6,000 to 15,000 milligrams of salt a day. None of these foodstuffs (fat, refined carbohydrates, and salt) are harmful in moderate amounts, but the SAD focuses on what should be the extras in our diet, slighting the vitamins, minerals, complex carbohydrates, fiber, and other elements we should be eating in large amounts. It is now to the point where we doctors spend much of our time trying to undo the harmful effects of unhealthful eating.

The Cancers of affluence

Clearly, fat flavors our food, but most authorities now agree that our high-fat SAD plays a large role in heart disease and many other problems, including cancer. Specifically, fat has been implicated as a causative factor in the *cancers of affluence*. The cancers of affluence are cancers of the breast, ovaries, and uterus in women; cancers of the prostate and pancreas in men; and cancers of the colon and rectum in men and women. I believe the cancers of affluence are responsible for at least 40 percent of cancer deaths in men and 60 percent in women— quite a price to pay for the "privilege" of eating the fatty SAD.

Remember, fat is both an initiator and promoter of cancer cells. Beyond a certain reasonable point, the more fat we eat, the greater the risk of developing prostate and other cancers.

The 4 ACES

In addition to cutting down on the amount of fat we eat, we can aid our doctors within in the fight against cancer and other diseases by making sure that our immune systems are as strong as possible.

Foods That Harm the Immune System

We should be consuming these substances only in small amounts:

Alcohol—Has been associated with cancer of the throat, gastrointestinal tract, liver, and more.

Salt—Eating large amounts of pickled foods is associated with increased cancer of the stomach.

Saccharin—Has been associated with cancer of the bladder.

Tobacco—Has been associated with cancer of the lungs, and more.

Fats—Fats may serve as both initiators and promoters of cancer. Avoid overeating *all* fatty foods, whether saturated or polyunsaturated; especially avoid fried foods.

Refined foods—Refined foods such as cakes, pies, candies, packaged cereals, and TV dinners are woefully short of nutrients. Not only that, all the sugar they contain robs us of some of the vitamins we get from other foods. Processed foods also tend to contain various artificial colors and other chemicals that do us no good.

Research has shown that the lack of even one vitamin or mineral can harm the immune system. Studies have also shown that certain vitamins, including the 4 ACES (vitamin A in the form of beta carotene, vitamin C, vitamin E, plus the mineral selenium), are especially helpful in the battle against cancer.

The 4 ACES fight cancer primarily in two ways: They are free-radical quenchers and antioxidants. Free radicals are natural by-products of body metabolism. Unfortunately, not everything made by the human body is beneficial. Free radicals are like little chain saws cutting through the body on a molecular level, damaging individual cells and the immune system, and increasing our risk of cancer. The 4 ACES (and other substances) help keep the free radicals under control. In their antioxidant capacity, the 4 ACES help guard against the dangers of oxidation (which can, if we stretch the imagination, be compared to the rusting of a piece of metal exposed to the air).

Vitamin A is found in fish liver oils, liver, milk, egg yolks, and other foods. Beta carotene, the plant form of vitamin A, is found in all green, yellow, and orange vegetables, and in most orange and yellow fruits. The beta carotene we get from our foods is not toxic—the body converts only as much as it needs. (Large doses of vitamin A in supplement form, however, may be toxic.) Vitamin C is found in asparagus, broccoli, brussels sprouts, cabbage, cantaloupe, citrus fruits, green beans, green peas, mangoes, and many other foods. Vitamin E is found in oils (such as vegetable oils), wheat germ, egg yolk, margarine, and legumes (peas, beans, and lentils). Selenium is found in garlic, onions, shellfish, red grapes, broccoli, whole wheat grains, chicken, and other foods. It is also present in vegetables, but the amount varies depending upon the amount in the soil where the vegetables were grown.

Another important prostate nutrient

Zinc is a most important mineral when it comes to prostate health. However, we Americans don't get enough zinc in our diets. In a study of Americans eating self-selected diets, 68 percent were found to have less than two-thirds of the RDA (recommended dietary allowance) for zinc, even though protein levels were sufficient.[1] Another study found 87 percent of 403 elderly people living in their own homes had zinc intakes in the low ranges.[2] A deficiency of zinc may be reflected in an enlarged prostate. However, often the only treatment needed to help shrink the prostate is additional zinc.

Crucifers against cancer

Foods known as "crucifers" are also potent allies of the doctor within. The crucifers are a family of vegetables named for what appears to be a cross in the flower, and include broccoli, brussels sprouts, cabbage, cauliflower, kohlrabi, kale, and bok choy. Eating crucifers encourages the formation of substances called *indoles* in our intestines. Studies have shown that indoles help to prevent certain cancers, including cancer of the colon.

The crucifers also contain cancer-fighting sulfides and sulforaphane, as well as good amounts of vitamin C, beta carotene, fiber, and complex carbohydrates, all of which are important soldiers in the war against disease. Eating crucifers has also been associated with a drop in the incidence of stomach and rectal cancer.

Other cancer-fighting foods

Garlic is one of my favorite cancer fighters because it works so well and tastes so good. Garlic's powers, once considered the stuff of fairy tales, are now being described in the medical literature. There are some 1,000 serious medical studies examining the health-boosting effects of garlic. We've known for years that garlic has antibiotic and antifungal properties that may be helpful in the battle against infections, including those of the prostate. We've also learned that it helps fight blood clots, thus lowering the risk of heart disease and stroke. More recently, it has been reported that garlic has strong anticancer properties as well. (There is no recommended daily dose of garlic, so I sprinkle it on many of my foods, use it crushed or minced in many of my recipes, and and also take Kyolic garlic capsules.)

Soy milk is another cancer fighter that works well and tastes great. People who drink soy milk have a substance called genistein in their urine. Research has shown that genistein helps to block the growth of any new capillaries that supply blood to tumors. Since developing tumors need an ever-increasing blood supply, preventing the growth of new capillaries may help stop tumors in their tracks. Many researchers and clinicians believe that the soy/genistein link may be the reason that Orientals, and Japanese in particular, have low rates of certain cancers, including those of the prostate and breast.

Soy foods, such as tofu, also contain a genistein. And the protease inhibitors found in soy foods (as well as in kidney beans, chickpeas, whole grains, and other foods) can prevent the conversion of normal cells to cancer cells in the early stages of cancer formation.

Garlic and soy foods are just two of the many delicious, health-giving foodstuffs that we can easily add to our diets.

Fresh vegetables, fruits, whole grains, peas, beans, and lentils

One of my patients told me that he had taken good notes during our discussions; he knew which foods to eat and which to avoid. "But let's face reality," he said. "I'm a single guy. I cook for myself or eat out a lot. I don't even know what's in most of my foods. Realistically, I'm not going to carry this list around and check everything I eat. Is there a simple way to know what's good for me?"

I tell my cancer (and other) patients to follow this simple rule: Eat four to six servings of fresh vegetables per day, plus fresh fruits, whole grains, peas, beans, and lentils, and consume plenty of water. Add small amounts of nonfat dairy products and fish. When eating mostly vegetables, fruits, whole grains, peas, beans, and lentils, one does not have to worry about the percent of saturated fat or polyunsaturated fat being taken in, because most of these foods are low in fat. (There are a few exceptions, such as avocados and coconuts, which are high in fat.) Neither do any of these foods have any cholesterol. (The simple rule for deciding which foods contain cholesterol is this: If the food came from an animal, it has cholesterol. If it grew in or from the ground, it does not.)

Accompany it all with plenty of fluids

Sitting under the bladder, the prostate is exposed to the toxins filtered out of the blood and placed into the urine by the kidneys. We should dilute this toxin-fluid with six to eight glasses of water per day. Also, eating vegetables is a good way to increase your water intake, for vegetables are 80 to 90 percent water. Cranberry juice is another

---

What to Eat: The Short and Simple List

The bulk of your diet should consist of fresh vegetables and fruits, whole grains, peas, beans, and lentils, including:

Apples	Collards	Papayas
Bananas	Garlic	Parsley
Beans (all kinds)	Ginger	Peaches
Broccoli	Kale	Pears
Brussels sprouts	Lentils	Peas (all kinds)
Cabbage	Mushrooms	Potatoes
Cantaloupe	Oat bran	Scallions
Carrots	Onions	Spinach
Cauliflower	Oranges	Whole grains (all kinds)

These are not the only foods you should be eating, but the list gives you an idea of the many great-tasting, healthful foods that are available. Be sure to eat a wide variety of foods, for no single food has all the nutrients necessary to keep a "doctor within" strong.

What to Drink

Water or cranberry juice—eight glasses a day.

---

helpful fluid to drink. Many doctors (including myself) have been prescribing cranberry juice for years to men with urinary and prostate problems. Now we know that the juice helps to prevent bacteria from adhering to the lining of the prostate and bladder.

Feeding your "doctor within": Putting it all together

In this section on the doctor within, several important elements have been drawn together to create a program of supplemental nutritional and dietary support. The plan has helped support conventional therapy for many of my prostate patients. Please remember that the support plan is meant to be used as an adjunct to other therapies, not as the sole therapy for prostate problems.

1. *Low-fat diet*—The standard American high-fat diet has been associated with cancer of the prostate and other problems. Many studies have shown that the high-fat diet is a burden on the immune system specifically, and on the body in general. I believe that a high-fat diet, especially one high in fat from beef, is a prime contributor to prostate cancer. If you have any problems with your prostate—or any other parts of the body—you can reduce the burden on your immune system by switching to a low-fat diet, eating mostly fresh vegetables, grains, and fruits, with small amounts of lean meat, low-fat dairy products, nuts, and seeds. It can't hurt, and many studies suggest it can help quite a bit.

2. *Two to three quarts of fluid a day, at least half of that being cranberry extract*—Drinking lots of water washes out any stagnant urine that has remained in the bladder, and it helps to "flush out the pipes." Studies in the *New England Journal of Medicine* in early 1994 showed that cranberry juice reduces lower urinary tract infections by interfering with the bacteria's ability to hold on to the cell walls in the lower urinary tract. Also, you should spread out your fluid intake over the course of the day. Do not drink an entire quart in one sitting. If possible, try to finish the bulk of your fluid intake by 4 P.M. in order to avoid excessive bathroom trips during the night.

3. *Antioxidants*—Taking these will often help control oxidation damage to the prostate and the rest of the body, and help to keep the immune system strong. This is what I generally recommend to my prostate patients, after having evaluated them thoroughly. The actual dosage for each patient can vary.

Vitamin A (beta carotene)—Begin with 25,000 IU twice a day, working up to 75,000 IU twice a day.

Vitamin C—Begin with 1,000 mg twice a day, working up to 4,000 mg twice a day.

Vitamin E—400 IU of d-alpha-tocopherol twice a day.

Selenium—100 micrograms once a day.

4. *Zinc, 30 mg daily*—The prostate contains about ten times more zinc than does any other organ. A lack of zinc has been associated with enlargement of the prostate, and some studies have shown that zinc helps reduce the swelling of chronic prostatitis. In one study, prostate size shrank in about 70 percent of the men taking zinc daily. Zinc is also helpful in dealing with BPH, sometimes completely solving the problem.

5. *DLPA*—The amino acid called DLPA (dl-phenylalanine) reduces pain by raising the endorphin levels. Endorphins are our natural, built-in painkillers and mood modulators, our "morphine within." More specifically, DLPA helps to protect the endorphins from endorphin-destroying enzymes in the body. DLPA has been shown to have not only endorphin-raising properties but also immune-boosting effects.[3] I often begin my patients with 750 mg of DLPA a day, but you should check with your doctor before taking the amino acid.[4]

6. *Plant products*—In Chapter 7, we discussed several plant products that have been used to help reduce swelling, pain, and other symptoms of prostate problems. These natural health aids include Prostat, saw palmetto, *Pygeum africanum*, *Equisetum arvense*, *Hydrangea arborescens*, and *Serenoa serrulata*.

A good diet and nutrition should be a part of every prostate treatment and prevention program—indeed, a part of everyone's healthy lifestyle. After all, good nutrition is vital for a strong immune system, and the immune system is our primary defense against cancer. Many patients have been helped by a good diet and potent nutritional support *plus* their regular medical/surgical treatment.

#3: Exercising Your Doctor Within

The prescription for a healthy doctor within also includes exercise. The cardiovascular benefits of exercise are well-known. As far as the immune system is concerned, exercise has been shown to reduce the incidence of many cancers, including those of the prostate and breast. Get out and walk thirty minutes a day, three to four days a week, or garden twenty minutes daily, or ride a bicycle or swim. The actual exercise is not as important as the fact that you are active, and, in addition, reasonable activity will help you to keep your weight under control.

Forget about fashion: The real reason for wanting to stay within your ideal weight range is that excess body fat is simply unhealthy. Obesity is a health risk. One study found that both men and women who were 25 percent or more overweight had an increased risk of rectal cancer, and males 25 percent or more overweight also had an increased risk of colon cancer. Another study of 750,000 men and women found an increase in cancer deaths in those who were 40 percent or more overweight.

IT MAKES SENSE

I urge all my male patients to adopt the four elements of the Healthy Prostate Program. There are no scientific studies proving that the program will prevent prostate problems, because it has never been subjected to large-scale, rigorous study. Each of the four elements, however, is a commonsense approach to serious problems. We can't always say what causes a certain disease, and we don't always know exactly how to cure it. But it is safe to say that self-awareness and regular checkups will help detect many ailments earlier than they would otherwise have been found. It's also safe to say that sexual smarts will reduce one's exposure to various sexually transmitted diseases and infections. And it's clear that high-fat diets are related to many cancers, including prostate cancer.

Finally, I can say with confidence that keeping your doctor within strong is an excellent defense against many diseases, including infections, cancers, and other problems caused by self-regulating systems that go haywire. With emphasis on all of its four elements, I believe that my Healthy Prostate Program is an excellent tool for all men to use in the fight against disease.

12

The Healthy Prostate Program, Part II: Treatment

We've already looked at the prostate, its diseases and the diagnosis of those diseases, plus the related tests, medicines, surgeries, and alternative therapies, plus aids to preventing prostate problems. Now it's time to put it all together. What should you and your doctor do if you have a prostate problem?

Back in medical school, we were taught that if you see a four-legged, long-tailed animal running by with a saddle on its back, it's probably a horse. Once in a very great while it'll be a zebra, but most of the time you'll be looking at a horse. Our teachers were trying to impress upon us the importance of beginning with the obvious when making a diagnosis and/or initiating treatment. Start with the most likely problems and solutions. Only if that doesn't work should we look for something more exotic. "Horses" first, then "zebras," if necessary.

The best horse approach is for the doctor to (1) carefully gather information by talking to the patient; (2) examine the entire patient, not just the prostate; (3) perform necessary tests; (4) rule out serious problems such as cancer; (5) handle the patient's pain or discomfort as necessary; and (6) begin treatment for the most likely problem. Obviously, the doctor should not spring to the most exotic (and expensive and dangerous) treatments, but rather should begin with the obvious.

WHO SHOULD TREAT PROSTATE PROBLEMS?

With most cases of BPH, prostatitis, or prostatodynia, you're best off appointing a good general doctor (such as your internist, general practitioner, or family practitioner) to begin, or at least oversee, your evaluation/treatment. Urologists are certainly qualified to handle these problems, but they should be used as expert consultants, not as primary-care physicians. Remember that urologists are trained to use strong medicines and to operate, so that's what they tend to do. And because you most likely do not meet the urologist until you have a urinary problem, this doctor probably doesn't know you, your family, and your desires as well as your primary-care physician does. That's why it's best to let your general doctor examine you in order to evaluate your condition and oversee your treatment.

If you have cancer, you may want to be examined and perhaps treated by cancer specialists and surgeons. If so, make sure that your general doctor oversees that treatment. Let the knowledgeable physician who knows you and cares about you, and who knows what all the others are doing, coordinate the many doctors who may become involved. I've seen too many cases go wrong because no single doctor was in charge, so I recommend that you have all the other doctors report back to your general doctor. Spend a lot of time talking with your general doctor after he's spoken with the other physicians and reviewed the results of all the tests. Use your general doctor, who is not wed to surgery or radiation or hormones, as a guide.

Let's look at my treatment approaches to prostatitis, prostatodynia, BPH, and prostate cancer.

The treatment outlines I present in this chapter are based upon my philosophy and my many years of experience in treating patients. I urge you to discuss all treatments with your physician. Insist that your doctor listen carefully to all of your symptoms and concerns. Learn all you can from your doctor, whether it be good news or bad. You and your doctor should be comfortable with the treatment program you decide upon, whether it be standard or alternative.

A Note on Medicines

Make sure your doctor tells you *why* he or she selected the prescribed medicine. Make the doctor justify the choice. Make sure your doctor asks you if you have allergies to specific medicines or to anything else, and what other medications you are taking. Mixing medicines can be dangerous, even deadly. Insist that your doctor review all of the side effects of the prescribed medicine with you. And make sure your doctor tells you how long he or she intends to keep you on the antibiotic; don't accept "we'll see" as an answer. *All* medicines are powerful and should be used in a carefully planned manner.

PROSTATITIS

Treatment Summary

Antibiotics (limited) to treat the immediate infection, antioxidants and other vitamins to strengthen the immune system and prevent further infections, zinc for the prostate, plenty of fluid, appropriate plant products, DLPA for pain, and a low-fat diet to help reduce the general burden on the body and immune system. This approach has been successful in 85 to 95 percent of my patients.

As you recall from Chapter 1, prostatitis is an inflammation of the prostate, usually caused by a bacterial infection. The problem can be chronic or acute, with symptoms ranging from the hardly noticeable to the very serious. The symptoms may come and go, or may hold steady. Bacteria may or may not be involved. Prostatitis can remain localized, or, in serious cases of acute prostatitis, the infection can spread to other parts of the body, leading to fever, chills, and other symptoms of a "full body" infection.

Treatment for Prostatitis, Round I

Once the diagnosis of prostatitis has been made, two questions must be asked: (1) Is there a bacterial invasion? and (2) Is the prostate inflamed? If the answer is yes to both questions, your doctor should begin the treatment. (If the answers are no, you may be dealing with another problem.) Treatment should consist of four steps:

Step 1. Antibiotics to treat the infection

The doctor can often prescribe an antibiotic on your first visit, before the results have come back from the laboratory. In general, I prefer starting with the older, less-dangerous, and less-expensive antibiotics. I look for the medicine that is most likely to help, that is least dangerous, and not so expensive that it turns the patient into a pauper.

Acute prostatitis is best treated with medicines that can build up high levels in the prostate, such as trimethoprim sulfamethoxazole. I generally start a patient on one of these medicines while waiting for the culture to return from the laboratory, and I may change the prescription when I see the lab results. As pointed out in Chapter 3, trimethoprim sulfamethoxazole medicines should be used carefully, for their side effects include skin rashes, bone marrow depression, allergic reactions, kidney failure, and other problems. Anyone sensitive to any form of sulfa, or anyone who has a folate deficiency, should avoid these medicines. If you develop any kind of skin rash or other new symptoms, stop the medicines immediately and call your doctor.

How long should this or a similar drug be taken? The truth is, we doctors don't really know. Some say two weeks, some prefer two months. I believe two weeks of medication is the maximum course that one should undergo for this condition. At that point, the doctor should reexamine the patient, take another culture, and reassess the situation. I don't always wait two weeks, of course. If the laboratory culture comes back in a few days and I can see that a better antibiotic is indicated, I will make the change immediately.

Results are often good with acute prostatitis. Chronic prostatitis, on the other hand, is more of a challenge. Somehow the infection has battled the immune system to a standstill and remains entrenched in the body. Since the problem has been around for a while and is not debilitating, the patient can usually wait three or four days for the culture and sensitivity[1] to return from the laboratory. When I see the results, I can select the medicine that would do the best job for that particular bacteria. Trimethoprim sulfamethoxazole is often a good medicine to start with because it can handle organisms usually found in the urinary tract, such as *E. coli, Klebsiella* species, *Enterobacter* species, and *Proteus mirabilis. Trimethoprim sulfamethoxazole should not be used in anyone allergic to sulfa, and it is possibly risky for people with any allergies.*

Erythromycin penetrates the prostate tissue well, and has a 30 to 40 percent success rate for chronic prostatitis six months after completion of therapy. (That is, the patients take the medicine for a few weeks, and when retested six months later, 30 to 40 percent are still infection free.) The most common adverse reactions to erythromycin include stomach cramping and discomfort, nausea, vomiting, and diarrhea.

Ciprofloxacin has been reported to have a 75 percent success rate three months after completion of therapy. A relatively new drug, ciprofloxacin works well against the most common bacteria found in urinary tract infections, such as *E. coli, Klebsiella pneumoniae, Enterobacter cloacae,* and *Proteus mirabilis. Some people have had serious reactions, including loss of consciousness, heart problems, sudden low blood pressure, rashes, fevers, even toxic hepatitis. This medicine should not be used by children or pregnant women.*

There are many other antibiotics that can be used for chronic prostatitis, depending upon the bacterial culture and your symptoms. (For more information on antibiotics, see Chapter 3.) Antibiotics may destroy the "good" bacteria in the body that protect against fungal infections, yeast overgrowth, and other problems. That's why it's important for people using antibiotics to protect themselves with probiotics, such as Lactobacillis and Bifidobacteria, that help to rebuild the body's supply of "good" bacteria.

Step 2. Supplemental nutritional and dietary support
(see Chapter 11).

Step 3. Checking for a hernia before beginning treatment

Actually, this should have been done during the initial examination, *before the diagnosis of prostatitis was made*, but it's often skipped.

Step 4. Screening for chlamydia and other sexually transmitted diseases

This is especially important with sexually active patients. Almost all sexually transmitted diseases can get into the prostate and produce symptoms that mimic those of prostatitis. Unfortunately, many doctors fail to check for sexually transmitted diseases.

At this point you should avoid:

1. Any X-ray imaging of the urinary tract, including the IVP discussed in Chapter 3. Even though it's popular and takes beautiful pictures, the IVP doesn't give the doctor essential information. The IVP mostly covers the upper urinary tract, not the prostate, so you get a lot of radiation in exchange for very little information. I've also seen patients who are allergic to iodine suffer serious complications from this test, including cardiac arrest. Unless you have other problems or complications, such as blood in the urine or a history of urinary tract stones, you should give the antibiotics, antioxidants, zinc, fluid, and plant products a chance to work before moving on to these potentially dangerous procedures.
2. Filling cystometry, also known as cystometrography or CMG. This invasive procedure is useful for evaluating patients with problems *after* prostate surgery, or in whom the doctor suspects neurologic problems. It's really not valuable at this time. (See Chapter 3 for more on CMG.)
3. Urethrocystoscopy. This procedure is useful for people undergoing surgery or balloon dilatation, but not for those suspected of

having an infection. Urethrocystoscopy can actually *cause* infections, plus bleeding, inability to urinate, and even death.

4. Any open-ended course of drug treatment, or treatment with multiple drugs. Insist that the doctor select medication carefully, with a specific objective and time line in mind.

You should return to your doctor's office in two weeks for a follow-up examination and discussion. At that time, your doctor should review all of your symptoms with you to see if the treatment is working, and should repeat the examination of your prostate.

If your symptoms have completely or mostly disappeared, you should stop taking antibiotics. However, you should continue with the appropriate plant products for an additional three to six weeks, and stay with the antioxidants, the zinc, and the fluid intake forever.

If your symptoms have not decreased satisfactorily, you and your doctor should move to Round II of treatment.

Treatment for Prostatitis, Round II

If you are still having symptoms of prostatitis after the first round of treatment, you may have either a very powerful bacterial infection, a nonbacterial infection, a problem with your immune system, or prostatodynia. Your doctor should check for all four possibilities:

Possibility 1: A very powerful bacterial infection

Such a bacterial infection may require a stronger dose of the medication that you've been taking, a longer course of treatment, or a different drug. I don't like to leave my patients on drugs indefinitely, hoping that a few more weeks or months of the medicine will handle the problem. You should continue with the drug therapy only if repeat laboratory tests show that the infection is still there, and if there is a reasonable chance that a stronger dose, a longer course of treatment, or a different drug will have the desired effect. Your doctor should check you out very carefully to make sure that you haven't suffered any serious side effects from the first round of treatment.

Possibility 2: A nonbacterial cause of infection

Your doctor began by looking for bacteria, because bacteria are the usual suspects in prostatitis. Now the search should be expanded to look for nonbacterial agents.

Possible nonbacterial causes of prostatitis include trichomonads protozoa, any kind of an injury to the urethra, as well as long-distance running and heavy lifting. It's difficult to make an exact diagnosis of prostatitis; all sorts of problems, affecting the area from the neck of the bladder down to the tip of the penis, can mimic the symptoms of prostatitis.

Possibility 3: An immune system problem

If an infection is not easily knocked out by the appropriate medicine, your doctor should ask why. The answer may be that your immune system is weak. With simple blood tests, your doctor can check your T cells, B cells, complements, and other aspects of your immune system. A weak immune system may have to be brought up to par before the prostatitis can be knocked out.

Possibility 4: Prostatodynia

When I was a young doctor, my older colleagues used to talk about prostatodynia, or what they called "strains." This was a vague diagnosis given to men who did heavy lifting at work or at home, who had pain in the groin area and/or symptoms of prostatitis, but who did not have a hernia or a prostate infection. Today we know that strains can be caused by damage to the pelvic floor muscles.

If the first round of treatment hasn't helped your prostatitis, your doctor should consider the possibility of a strain, even if a hernia has been ruled out. I've successfully treated many cases of "prostatitis" with nonsteroidal anti-inflammatories, DLPA, and rest.

If your symptoms have not improved much after Round II, you and your doctor should move to Round III.

Treatment for Prostatitis, Round III

Round II included continued or additional medications, as well as a search for and treatment of nonbacterial agents, a weakened immune system, and/or a "strain." If Rounds I and II haven't significantly reduced your inflammation and symptoms, you may not really have prostatitis. (Now it's time to start looking for "zebras.")

Prostatitis can be confused with BPH, a bladder infection, a urethral infection, and even cancer of the prostate. Further diagnostic studies, possibly followed by cystoscopy, are now indicated.

Always remember: "horses before zebras." *Every single medicine, test, procedure, and surgery is risky to some degree. If you don't need it, skip it.* And if your history, physical examination, and routine tests suggest prostatitis, opt for the obvious, conservative treatment (unless there's reason to suspect a more serious problem).

PROSTATODYNIA

Treatment Summary

Pain medication as necessary, plus DLPA, antioxidants and other vitamins, zinc, fluids, plant products, and a low-fat diet to reduce symptoms while you and your doctor search for the underlying cause.

Prostatodynia is pain that comes from the prostate, or the area of the prostate. Prostatodynia may be caused by an inflammation of the muscles of the pelvic floor, a stricture or spasm of the urethra, or bladder neck sclerosis. The underlying problem could be prostatitis, extensive prostate calcification, or even prostate cancer. Prostatodynia may also be associated with marathon running or bicycling, long-distance driving, or weight lifting. Many patients with prostatodynia also have back pain or other back problems. Interstitial cystitis, various anal and rectal problems, and/or bladder cancer may also be the cause. The diagnosis of prostatodynia is a "wastebasket" diagnosis, one we doctors give when we're not sure what the problem may be. The patient's pain is real; it may come and go, it may be an aching, a coldness, or an itchy sensation. The testicles and rectum may be involved, and there may be pain upon urinating or ejaculating. Treatment for prostatodynia consists of:

1. Pain medication, if necessary. Nonsteroidal anti-inflammatories are often helpful.
2. A continued search for the underlying problem.
3. Prostat (see page 124). I've had great success by prescribing it.
4. Supplemental nutritional and dietary support (see Chapter 11).

At this point you should avoid any X-ray imaging of the urinary tract, including the IVP, unless you have other problems or complications; filling cystometry; urethrocystoscopy; and any open-ended course of drug treatment, or treatment with multiple drugs.

Again, remember "horses before zebras." *Every single medicine, test, procedure, and surgery is risky to some degree. If you don't need it, skip it.* If your history, physical examination, and routine tests suggest prostatodynia, opt for the obvious, conservative treatment (unless there's reason to suspect a more serious problem).

BENIGN PROSTATIC HYPERTROPHY (BPH)

Treatment Summary

Several options are available, depending upon the severity of your symptoms, your doctor's findings, and your general health and lifestyle. If possible, I recommend beginning with "watchful waiting." The next step is to use noninvasive alternative means, then medications, and finally surgery, if necessary.

BPH is a benign condition in which the prostate enlarges. It happens in almost all men as they age. BPH can go entirely unnoticed, or cause serious problems. In some cases the patient improves without any help whatsoever, while others require aggressive treatment. BPH is a puzzling problem because the size of the prostate is not necessarily related to the symptoms. You can have a greatly enlarged prostate, but no symptoms. On the other hand, a relatively small prostate that squeezes the urethra can cause a great deal of difficulty. Many cases of BPH improve without any treatment; time is their cure. On the other hand, some cases may progress to urinary tract infections, a complete inability to urinate, kidney damage, and/or other problems.

There are three main standard approaches to treating BPH:

1. Watchful waiting—Keeping an eye on the situation with your doctor, discussing potential problems and possible outcomes.
2. Medical treatment—Medicines to treat the various symptoms and/or shrink the enlarged prostate.
3. Surgery and invasive procedures—Options ranging from lasers to complete removal of the prostate.

The approach that is best for you depends upon your situation. How large is your prostate? Does it have the normal "feel"? Is it boggy (soft and squishy)? Is it covered with nodes? What are your symptoms? Do they bother you? Have they become worse with time? Do you have an infection?

Let's imagine four typical BPH scenarios. Before you start reading the scenarios, review the American Urological BPH Symptom Index you filled out in Chapter 2.

Scenario #1. On routine examination, the doctor discovers that you have an enlarged prostate, but there are no nodes on the prostate and you have no symptoms of BPH.

If your prostate is enlarged but you have no symptoms, no nodes, and there are no other signs of danger, "watchful waiting" is the best treatment. A good number of men with BPH will go to their graves without ever experiencing any symptoms. "Watchful waiting" consists of:

1. **Discussion**—You and your doctor discuss the prostate, BPH, and possible future problems.
2. **Examination**—Your doctor performs a complete physical and orders laboratory studies, including a DRE and PSA, yearly. If the DRE or PSA is suspicious or elevated, a transrectal ultrasound will help rule out cancer.
3. **Reevaluation**—You are reevaluated at least once a year, or more often if you're concerned.
4. **Risk factors**—If you have other risk factors for cancer (e.g., if you're an adult black male, if you're a white male over the age of 60, if you eat a high-fat diet, or if you smoke cigarettes), your doctor carefully considers checking you for cancer.

At this point you should avoid any X-ray imaging of the urinary tract, including the IVP, unless you have other problems or complications; filling cystometry; urethrocystoscopy; and any open-ended course of drug treatment, or treatment with multiple drugs. *Every single medicine, test, procedure, and surgery is risky to some degree. If you don't need it, skip it.* If your history, physical examination, and routine tests suggest BPH, opt for the obvious, conservative treatment (unless there's reason to suspect a more serious problem). BPH often gets better on its own, without treatment. But don't forget the "watchful" part of "watchful waiting," for the condition may grow worse.

Scenario #2. You have mild symptoms and, during a routine examination, the doctor discovers that you have an enlarged prostate.

If you have an enlarged prostate and some mild symptoms, I recommend "watchful waiting" combined with:

1. **Supplemental nutritional and dietary support** (see Chapter 11).
2. **Lifestyle changes**—An example would be drinking less or no liquids before going to bed.
3. **Changes in your prescription and nonprescription medications**—Certain cold and sinus medicines that you can buy in the

drugstore can make prostate problems worse. So can prescription medications such as Donnatal, which interferes with the proper emptying of the bladder, and other medications. *Discuss all of your prescription and nonprescription medicines with your physician and your pharmacist.*

4. **PSA testing**—Even if you are only forty years old, you should have a PSA test. If it's low, there's no problem; just keep your eye on it. If the PSA is high, you should have a transrectal ultrasound with a biopsy of anything that looks cancerous.

5. **A discussion of medical and surgical options**—This is to inform you should such options become necessary in the future.

At this point you should avoid any X-ray imaging of the urinary tract, including the IVP, unless you have other problems or complications; filling cystometry; urethrocystoscopy; and any open-ended course of drug treatment, or treatment with multiple drugs. *Every single medicine, test, procedure, and surgery is risky to some degree. If you don't need it, skip it.*

Scenario #3. You have mild to moderate symptoms of BPH, enough to concern you, and your doctor makes a diagnosis of BPH.

Very careful "watchful waiting" is still possible, but at this stage most patients are troubled by urinary and other difficulties. They generally want something done, and with good reason. There are two new options at this stage: medication and surgery. I generally recommend medicine before surgery, preferring to save the knife for last, unless it's absolutely necessary. Should you have mild to moderate symptoms that concern you, and should your doctor make the diagnosis of BPH, I suggest:

1. **A discussion of the situation.**
2. **The appropriate plant products, generally including Prostat**—If they don't work, I go on to the medical therapy in step 5.
3. **Medicines to relieve symptoms, if necessary.**
4. **Supplemental nutritional and dietary support** (see Chapter 11).
5. **Medical therapy**—This would involve alpha blockers or Proscar, but only if necessary, and only after careful discussion of the pros and cons with your physician.
6. **A discussion of future surgical and other options.**

Let's take a brief look at medicines that would be employed in steps 3 and 5. (For more complete discussion of prostate medications, see Chapter 4.) The alpha-blocking drugs such as Hytrin, Minipress, and Cardura help by relaxing the smooth muscle of the prostate and bladder neck. They are also used to treat high blood pressure. Many patients using the alpha blockers have reported a perceptible, albeit small, improvement in symptoms. Unfortunately, the use of alpha blockers for BPH is relatively new, so we don't know what the long-term benefits—or risks—will be. Although the alpha blockers help to relieve the symptoms, there is so far no evidence that the drugs will actually reduce the incidence of BPH complications or eliminate any eventual need for surgery. Alpha-blocking drugs have many side effects, so the dosage must be carefully monitored, starting on the low side and working up. Also, your blood pressure must be checked regularly because of the role of the alpha blockers in lowering blood pressure.

The newly approved drug Proscar has also shown some promise in early studies. While alpha blockers make smooth muscle in the prostate relax, Proscar is designed to actually shrink the prostate. Because it is relatively new, we don't know how useful or dangerous it may be in the long run. And even if Proscar does shrink the prostate, there is no guarantee that the shrinkage will relieve all or most of the symptoms. Proscar's side effects include ejaculatory dysfunction, impotence, and a decreased interest in sex. Proscar can also decrease serum PSA levels by up to 50 percent, making it harder for your doctor to check for cancer. Because of the side effects and the long course of treatment necessary, the dosage for Proscar must be carefully monitored, starting on the low side and working up. And you may need to take Proscar for six or more months before determining whether it will work for you.

There are also medicines that will help relieve some of the pain and discomfort of BPH, although they do not deal with the root problem. I've used nonsteroidal, anti-inflammatory medications such as ketoprofen, ibuprofen, and flurbiprofen. I always use the medications with caution, however, and only when necessary and for a limited period of time. These medications must be taken on a full stomach to prevent ulcers, stomach irritation, or bleeding. I've also found that DLPA is very helpful in reducing the pain that may be associated with BPH, but not the inflammation.

Make sure your doctor tells you why he or she selected the medicine prescribed, reviews all the possible side effects, and tells you how long you are expected to remain on the medicine. Make sure the doctor asks about all of your allergies and which other medicines, supplements, or other substances you are taking.

Scenario #4. *You have moderate to severe symptoms of BPH, enough to interfere with your lifestyle and to worry you, and your doctor makes a diagnosis of BPH.*

The BPH has made your life uncomfortable, and you may be at risk for bladder or kidney damage, recurrent urinary tract infections, serious amounts of blood in the urine, and other problems. Medication is still a viable option, but you and your doctor must seriously consider surgery and other invasive procedures, ranging from balloon dilatation to complete removal of the prostate. At this point I suggest:

1. **A trial therapy with plant products.**
2. **Medicines to relieve symptoms, as necessary.**
3. **Supplemental nutritional and dietary support** (see Chapter 11).
4. **Medical therapy with alpha blockers or Proscar**—Take this step if both you and your doctor feel it is necessary.
5. **Surgical or other procedures**—Take this step if both you and your doctor agree that it is necessary.

PROSTATE CANCER

Treatment Summary

Treatments include radiation, hormone therapy, and completely removing the prostate. Although removal of the prostate and radiation have helped some men, they have not been fully tested, and have serious side effects. For many men, especially those in their seventies, "watchful waiting" is a good option.

Prostate cancer is a major cancer in men, striking some 200,000 and killing 38,000 men yearly. Deciding what to do when you have prostate cancer is difficult and emotionally charged, for cancer is frightening. However, I remind my patients that even though many men will eventually develop cancer of the prostate, odds are that they will never know they have it and will die of something else. The great danger is that the cancer will slip out of the prostate and move to other parts of the body. Unfortunately, we can't tell which tumors will spread—and by the time they migrate, it's too late to stop them.

Frightened by the possibility that their cancer will spread and become deadly, 24,000 men opt for surgery every year. Thousands more ask for radiation or hormone therapy, and an unknown number try cryosurgery, hyperthermia, and/or various alternative therapies.

Surgery, radiation, and hormone therapy are all aggressive—but often dangerous—approaches to a sometimes aggressive, dangerous disease. But many studies suggest that doing nothing—"watchful waiting"—can be almost as effective for certain men. The Prostate Patient Outcomes Research Team has devised a computer model that shows a sixty-year-old man with moderately aggressive cancer and an excellent doctor. If he undergoes surgery with minimal complications, he should live approximately seventeen more years. But if the same man opts for "watchful waiting," he should live approximately sixteen more years, without the discomfort, risks, or side effects of surgery.

Here are the general guidelines I present to my patients to help them decide what to do if they have prostate cancer.

If the Cancer Is Confined to the Prostate and Is Not Palpable

"Watchful waiting" is a cautious option, especially for men in their late sixties or older. I stress to the men, however, that no one can predict the course of their cancer. As part of the "watchful waiting" program, I suggest:

1. **Regular examinations**—Keep a very careful eye on the man's general health. Repeated DREs, PSAs, ultrasounds with biopsies, and other tests should be carefully monitored for any signs of change.
2. **Supplemental nutritional and dietary support** (see Chapter 11).
3. **Lifestyle changes.**
4. **A careful check of all prescription and nonprescription medications**—Certain cold and sinus medicines bought in the drugstore can make prostate problems worse. So can ulcer and other prescription medications such as Donnatol, which interferes with the proper emptying of the bladder. *Discuss all your prescription and nonprescription medicines with your physician and your pharmacist.*

I recommend that men go to a prostate cancer support group and talk to those who have already made their choices, and that they learn as much as possible about prostate cancer and all the treatment options.

If the Cancer Is Confined to the Prostate and Is Palpable

"Watchful waiting" is still a very cautious possibility, especially for men in their late sixties or older. But the decision to watch and wait should be made very carefully for each man, with doctor and patient discussing and deciding together. For younger men, a radical prostatectomy to remove the prostate before any cancerous cells have spread should be carefully considered by both doctor and patient. If it's possible to pluck the entire thing out and be done with it forever, the risks of surgery may be worth facing. However, the risks of radical prostatectomy include impotence in 30 to 70 percent of patients, a constricted urine flow in 10 percent, incontinence in 6 percent, injury to the rectum in 3 percent, and death in 1 percent. And remember that about 90 percent of the time, the surgery gets all of the cancer out of the patient's body, but 10 percent of the time, it leaves something behind. Seek out men who have already undergone surgery, radiation, hormone therapy, and other approaches. Talk to them, learn from them. Investigate all of the conventional and alternative therapies before making a decision. Supplemental nutritional and dietary support can be a helpful adjunct to therapy.

If the Cancer Has Spread Beyond the Prostate

Now we're into a whole new realm of treatment. You and your doctor must consider the various passive and aggressive options for treating this cancer, just as you would if you were faced with any other cancer that has spread. Seek out men who have already undergone surgery, radiation, hormone therapy, and other approaches. Talk to them, learn from them. Investigate all the conventional and alternative therapies before making a decision. As with other stages, supplemental nutritional and dietary support can be a helpful adjunct to therapy. This would be a good time for your doctor to work with a physician trained in alternative therapies. Many men do remarkably well with a combination of both standard and alternative methods.

What the Major Cancer Organizations Recommend

National Cancer Institute

These are the National Cancer Institute's recommendations as of January 29, 1994. They are based on the A, B, C cancer staging system described in Chapter 8.

Stage A1—For younger men, radical prostatectomy or external radiation is recommended. "Watchful waiting" is an option for older men with slow-growing cancer and no symptoms.

Stage A2—External radiation therapy, internal radiation therapy (usually in conjunction with dissection of the pelvic lymph node), radical prostatectomy, and cryosurgery are options. For older men and those with another, more serious illness, "watchful waiting."

Stage B—Options include radical prostatectomy, probably with dissection of the pelvic lymph node, often followed by radiation surgery; external radiation therapy; internal radiation therapy, often with dissection of the pelvic lymph node; cryosurgery. For older men and those with another, more serious illness, "watchful waiting."

Stage C—Options include radical prostatectomy, probably with dissection of the pelvic lymph nodes, often followed by radiation surgery; external radiation therapy; and internal radiation therapy, often with dissection of the pelvic lymph node. For those unable to have surgery or radiation therapy, treatment options include radiation therapy geared toward relieving symptoms, transurethral resection, and hormone therapy. For older men and those with another, more serious illness, "watchful waiting."

Stage D1—Options include external radiation therapy, possibly in conjunction with hormone therapy; radical prostatectomy with orchiectomy; and hormone therapy. For older men and those with another, more serious illness, "watchful waiting."

Stage D2—Options include hormone therapy, external beam radiation therapy to relieve symptoms, transurethral resection, chemotherapy, and radiation.

Recurrent Prostate Cancer—Options vary. If you've already had your prostate removed and the cancer comes back, radiation therapy is an option. If the cancer has spread to other parts of the body, hormone therapy is likely. Radiation therapy may be used to relieve symptoms. Chemotherapy may be used.

The National Cancer Institute recommendations are well in keeping with the traditional, aggressive beliefs of the medical establishment. Action is preferred to inaction.

American Cancer Society

Here is the American Cancer Society's discussion of treatment for prostate cancer, as presented in their Cancer Response System, Number 462557.

Surgery—Cancers confined to the prostate are usually successfully handled by a total prostatectomy. Nerve damage leading to erectile and urinary difficulties is common.

Radiation—Cancers confined to the prostate, or that have only spread to nearby tissue, can be cured by internal or external radiation. In later stages of the cancer, radiation may be used to relieve symptoms, but not to cure. Impotency is a common side effect.

Hormone Treatment—Useful for cancers that have spread, or recurring prostate cancer. Not beneficial if used *before* symptoms occur.

Chemotherapy—Can slow tumor growth and reduce pain and other symptoms in advanced cases, but it does not cure the cancer. Side effects include anemia, increased risk of infections and mouth sores, immune system depression, nausea, vomiting, and hair loss.

Cryosurgery—Considered experimental as of March 1994.

There are no hard-and-fast answers to the treatment question, for medicine is as much an art as it is a science. However, there is a philosophy of treatment: "Horses before zebras"—the least damaging treatment before the more dangerous, with the patient's welfare and concerns carefully considered.

An "Official" Look at the Risks of Some Treatments

Here's a listing of some of the risks that one faces when undergoing surgery, radiation, or hormonal therapy for prostate cancer. I've adapted this listing from a larger one presented by William J. Catalona, M.D., in the *New England Journal of Medicine*.[2] I don't necessarily agree with the "risk percentages" that he presents, but I use them here because of the considerable controversy over numbers.

Radical Prostatectomy

Blood loss during surgery (1–2 liters)
Impotence (30–60%)
Urinary incontinence (5–15%)
Thromboembolism (1–12%)
Vesicourethral anastomotic stricture (0.6–25%)
Wound infection (0.4–16%)
Myocardial infarction (heart attack) (0.4%)
Death (0.1–2%)
Rectal injury (0.1–7%)
Urethral injury (0.1–0.3%)
Postoperative bleeding (0.1%)

Radiation: External Beam

Impotence (40–60%)
Acute proctitis, cystitis, urinary retention, penoscrotal edema (30–50%)
Chronic cystitis (8%)
Urethral stricture (4%)
Chronic enteritis (3%)
Chronic proctitis (2%)
Chronic diarrhea (less than 1%)
Chronic edema (less than 1%)
Incontinence (less than 1%)
Death (less than 0.1%)

(continued)

(Continued from previous page)

Radiation: Interstitial	During surgery: hemorrhage Shortly after surgery: pelvic abscess, lymphocele, wound infection, hematoma, thrombophlebitis, pulmonary embolism, urinary retention, urinary fistula, pelvic-nerve palsy
Hormone Therapy: Orchiectomy	Hot flashes, decreased libido, decreased sexual potency, wound hematoma or infection
Hormone Therapy: DES[3]	Gynecomastia (breast enlargement), thromboembolism, fluid retention, gastrointestinal upset, decreased libido (sexual drive), decreased sexual potency
Hormone Therapy: LHRH[4]	Decreased libido, decreased sexual potency, hot flashes
Hormone Therapy: Flutamide[5]	Gynecomastia, nausea, diarrhea, hepatoxicity.

I've had considerable success treating prostatitis, prostatodynia, and BPH *without* drugs and surgery, or with just enough medicines to "get over the hump." The overwhelming majority of men do not have to—and should not—remain on medication for long periods of time. And I've also seen some cancer patients do well even though they bypassed the traditional approaches.

Remember: The doctor is not God and does not have all the answers. However, the best doctor will have a lot of information, experience, and wisdom from which you can draw when making your choices.

13

The Latest Word on Treating the Prostate

As of this writing, the latest word on treating BPH (benign prostatic hypertrophy) comes from an article in the very prestigious *New England Journal of Medicine*.[1] The author of the paper notes that TURP (transurethral resection of the prostate), the preferred treatment for BPH, is losing some of its luster. New studies are suggesting that it's not the definitive surgery it was once hoped to be. Besides the various postsurgical complications, 15 to 20 percent of men undergoing the TURP will eventually need a new surgery. Another interesting finding from preliminary studies is that men who have had TURP actually have a shorter life expectancy than those who have had a radical prostatectomy. This is an odd finding, for you would expect those who had TURP, the "lesser" surgery, to do better over the long run than those who underwent radical surgery.

As more doubts are raised about the surgery for BPH, medicines are increasingly being praised. If surgeries are used less and medicines more, the responsibility for caring for men with BPH will shift away from the urologists/surgeons and toward internists and other primary care physicians.

Cryosurgery received a boost during a report to the Radiological Society of North America delivered by Dr. Giovanna Casola of the University of California, San Diego, Medical Center.[2] Dr. Casola reported on some 300 men who underwent cryosurgery for prostate cancer, most in Stage A or B. When about half of the patients were rebiopsied three to six months later, some 85 percent of them had negative results (no cancer was detected).

As for the BPH medicines, the article reports that Proscar (finesteride) is "only moderately effective in treating symptomatic" BPH.[3] Hytrin (terazosin) and related drugs continue to show promise, but none has yet emerged as the "silver bullet" against BPH.

221

Meanwhile, researchers are refining our ability to detect prostate cancer, as well as our ability to determine whether or not a particular cancer should be treated or can be carefully watched. Two studies in the journal *Cancer* suggest that PSA density "is useful in discriminating prostate cancer in men with normal digital rectal examinations and borderline PSA levels. . . ."[4] In other words, PSA density can be a decisive determining factor in many borderline cases. PSA density, rather than the simple PSA, is also a better tool for predicting which patients are likely to suffer from a regrowth of prostate cancer following surgery.

On the high-tech front, a team headed by Dr. Jeffrey Ross, chief of pathology at Albany Medical College, has reported on the use of DNA analysis to determine whether or not a man should have surgery, should he develop prostate cancer.[5] Using ultrasound, a biopsy of the cancer can be taken and the tissue's DNA analyzed. The study's authors feel that DNA analysis will spare men the pain of unnecessary surgery should their prostate cancer be aggressive and highly likely to recur even after a radical prostatectomy.

THE FUTURE LOOKS GREAT

Having been treating patients for forty years, I am truly excited and enthusiastic about the future of prostate health. Great scientific advances are being made; new ideas such as freezing and heating troubled prostates are being tested. Forty years ago, the treatment for prostatitis consisted of a prostatic massage. I remember doing that, and having the patients say, "Can't you use your little finger?" Forty years ago, the treatment for BPH was to do nothing, or to operate. Back then, doctors put metal tubes we called "sounds" into the tip of the penis, pushing them up into the urethra in order to break up scar formation caused by gonorrhea and other diseases. I hated to do that; it was the most painful procedure I had to perform on a patient who was awake. Today, happily, we can cure so many more problems thanks to great advances in preventing and treating infections.

All good doctors would agree that preventing disease is much better than having to treat it. Safe sex, or abstinence until marriage, can go a long way toward preventing much prostatitis. Most every man who comes to see me complaining of the symptoms of a prostate infection has recently had unprotected sex with someone he just met. Simple measures, like abstinence or having only protected sex, are great preventives.

Another very powerful preventive measure is keeping the immune system as strong as possible. A strong doctor within will block almost all infections that try to gain a foothold in your body.

There's even great news on the prostate cancer front. We're not really that good at treating it, but I believe that we can prevent most cases of prostate cancer. For years, I've called prostate cancer one of the "cancers of affluence," a cancer associated with the high-fat, high-animal-protein diet we eat in North America and Europe. The incidence of prostate cancer is much lower in countries where the diet is low-fat, with moderate amounts of animal protein. This simple fact offers us a risk-free approach to preventing prostate cancer. The low-fat diet is already being recommended highly by the government, the National Institutes of Health, and others as a means of lowering the risk of coronary artery disease and cancer in general. We're already headed in that direction: Better prostate health is bound to be a beneficial side effect of the movement toward more healthful eating.

The use of antioxidants and the program described in Chapter 11 is a highly valid approach to preventing *all* cancers, especially the cancers of affluence. A major study of 22,000 doctors has shown that those taking in the highest amounts of beta carotene had only 12 percent of the expected cancers. Many other studies are showing how the antioxidants help us resist cancer by opposing and destroying free radicals and preventing oxidation. This news offers us another strong weapon to use against cancer.

Even the very conservative National Cancer Institute, which is practically an enemy of alternative medicine, believes we can prevent many cancers simply by changing our diets. The institute is spending millions of dollars to convince the American public to eat more vegetables and fruits, having finally realized that the various vitamins, phytochemicals, and other substances in fruits, vegetables, grains, peas, beans, and lentils help protect us against cancer. Surgery and radiation haven't won the war against cancer: Broccoli and carrots may be our best weapons.

I sincerely believe that the Healthy Prostate Program goes a long way toward reducing the risk of prostatitis and prostate cancer, and that it is helpful in relieving many of the symptoms of BPH. I believe that most men, working with their physicians, can enjoy great prostate health. And the side effects of the Healthy Prostate Program will be better overall health as well. If you follow the Program carefully, you'll be on your way to living young and healthy, to a very old age.

Appendix

SOURCES FOR MORE INFORMATION

Cancer and Urologic Information Resources

American Foundation for Urologic Disease
300 W. Pratt St., Suite 401, Baltimore, MD 21201
(800) 242-2383

According to the foundation's Mission Statement, it is "dedicated to the prevention and cure of urologic diseases through the expansion of medical research and the education of the public and health care professionals concerning urologic diseases and dysfunction." The foundation publishes a quarterly newsletter, sends out information upon request, and serves as an international clearinghouse for more than 300 prostate cancer support groups.

CancerFax®
(301) 402-5874

CancerFax® is a simple, fast way to get information about cancer from the National Cancer Institute's Physician Data Query (PDQ) system. You must contact the number above via a fax machine, and punch the appropriate keys to request information.

Cancer Information Service (CIS)
(800) 4-CANCER, or (800) 422-6237

CIS provides accurate, up-to-date information on cancer to patients and their families, to health professionals, and to the general public. Call to get information on the latest cancer treatments and clinical trials, tips on how to detect cancer in its early stages, tips on how to reduce your risk of cancer, and details of community services for patients and their families. All calls are confidential. Spanish-speaking staff members are available. Free booklets on cancer can be ordered. CIS serves the entire United States and Puerto Rico between 9 A.M. and 7 P.M. (local time) Monday through Friday. CIS is sponsored by the National Cancer Institute.

Help for Incontinent People (HIP)
(800) BLADDER

HIP is a leading source of advocacy, education, and information about the causes, treatments, and management options for incontinence. It offers a variety of printed and audiovisual programs. HIP is a national, nonprofit organization.

The Matthews Foundation for Prostate Cancer Research
1010 Hurley Way, Suite 195, Sacramento, CA 95825
(800) 234-6284

The Matthews Foundation is dedicated to reducing the suffering caused by prostate cancer by helping to increase public awareness, education outreach, and funding of research into the causes, prevention, and treatment of the disease. Through its toll-free hotline, the foundation provides information to over 1,000 callers monthly. Free educational literature is available from the foundation, which also lends books and videotapes.

National Cancer Institute
Office of Cancer Communication, Building 31, Room 10A24,
9000 Rockville Pike, Bethesda, MD 20892
(800) 4-CANCER

The National Coalition for Cancer Survivorship (NCCS)
(301) 650-9127

NCCS is the largest network of independent organizations and individuals working in the area of cancer support, advocacy, and survivorship. NCCS's goal is to generate a nationwide awareness of survivorship, emphasizing that one can have a vibrant, productive life after the diagnosis of cancer. NCCS facilitates communication among those involved with cancer, serves as a clearinghouse for information and materials on survivorship, advocates the interests of cancer survivors to legislators, assists in cases of employment discrimination, and promotes the study of survivorship research. NCCS's quarterly newsletter, *Networker*, offers survivorship news, feature articles, interviews, and book reviews.

Patient Advocates for Advanced Cancer Treatments (PAACT)
1143 Parmelee, N.W., Grand Rapids, MI 49504
(616) 453-1477

PAACT engages in research from databases, medical journals, clinical trials, published and unpublished medical papers, and its own patient registry in order to obtain the latest and most up-to-date information on the detection, diagnosis, evaluation, and treatment of prostate cancer. This information is made available through PAACT's newsletter, *Cancer Communication,* and through other books and pamphlets.

Prostate Cancer Support Network
(410) 727-2908

The network is sponsored by the American Foundation for Urologic Disease (see above).

US TOO
300 W. Pratt St., Suite 401, Baltimore, MD 21201
(800) 808-7866, or (708) 323-1002

US TOO is dedicated to helping prostate cancer survivors and their families lead healthy and productive lives. US TOO provides fellowship, counseling, discussion, and information on the latest medical options for prostate cancer. US TOO publishes a monthly international newsletter containing articles from medical experts and cancer survivors, and has over two hundred support groups in the United States, Canada, and Turkey.

The Wellness Community
2716 Ocean Park Blvd., Suite 1040, Santa Monica, CA 90405-5211
(310) 314-2555

The Wellness Community is the largest U.S. support program providing free psychological and emotional support to cancer patients and their families. The many Wellness Communities throughout the United States offer support groups, educational materials, and other services. Contact national headquarters to find a center near you.

There are many, many other local support and information groups. If you would like to find a local support group but don't know how, call the groups above, or ask your doctor.

Notes

1 The Prostate—An Overview of the "Unknown" Gland

1. This information is taken from Main, Henry. *The Story Behind the Words*. Springfield, IL: Charles C Thomas; 1958. See pages 228 and 309.

2 What Can Go Wrong—and Why

1. Berry SJ, Coffey DS, Walsh PC, Ewing LL. The development of human benign prostatic hyperplasia with age. *J Urol.* 1984;132:474–479.

2. Silverberg E, Boring CC, Squires TS. Cancer statistics, 1990. *CA.* 1990; 40:9–26; Scott R Jr, Mutchnik DL, Laskowski TZ, Schmalhorst WR. Carcinoma of the prostate in elderly men: incidence, growth characteristics and clinical significance. *J Urol.* 1969;101:602–607; Montie JE, Wood DP Jr, Pontes JE, Boyett JM, Levin HS. Adenocarcinoma of the prostate in cysto-prostatectomy specimens removed for bladder cancer. *Cancer.* 1989;63: 381–385.

3. Murphy GP, et al. The national survey of cancer in the United States by the American College of Surgeons. *J Urol.* 1982;127:928–934.

4. Prostate cancer may be linked to genetic defect. Charlene Laino. *Medical Tribune.* December 15, 1994, p 1. See also the *Los Angeles Times*'s report on the study, Prostate cancer may have roots in genetic defect, *Los Angeles Times.* November 22, 1994, p A30.

5. Moul JW. Prostatitis. Sorting out the different causes. *Postgraduate Medicine.* October 1993: 94 (5).

6. Moul JW, ibid.

3 How Prostate Problems Are Diagnosed

1. As reported by Wickens, Barbara. Middle-age suffering. *Maclean's.* March 16, 1992, p 45.

2. Abstracts. *Geriatrics*. July 1994: 49 (7): 52, notes that "using finesteride for BPH can decrease PSA by 50% after 6 to 12 months of treatment. . . ."

3. Osterling JE. Prostate specific antigen: improving its ability to diagnose early prostate cancer. *JAMA*. 1992;267(16):2236–2238.

4. Yuan, JY, et al. Effects of rectal examination, prostatic massage, ultrasonography and needle biopsy on serum prostate specific antigen levels. As reported in the "Domestic abstracts." *JAMA*. 1992;268:188.

5. Another study found that "No clinically important effects on serum PSA levels were noted after DRE." Drawford ED, et al. The effect of digital rectal examination on prostate-specific antigen levels. *JAMA*. 1992;267: 2227–2228.

6. *The Medical Herald*. July 1994, p 27.

7. I am indebted to Michael Krane, M.D., Medical Director of RadNet Management, Inc., in Los Angeles, for information about the use of bone scans and MRIs for prostate problems.

4 Medicines for the Prostate

1. Adapted from Benign Prostatic Hyperplasia: Diagnosis and Treatment. Quick Reference Guide for Clinicians. Number 8. U.S. Department of Health and Human Services, Public Health Service, Agency for Health Care Policy and Research. AHCPR Publication No. 94-0583. February 1994. Rockville, MD.

5 Surgeries for the Prostate

1. Lu-Yao GL, et al. An assessment of radical prostatectomy. *JAMA*. May 26, 1993;20:2634–2636.

2. Ibid.

3. I'd like to thank Douglas Chinn, M.D., of the Alhambra Hospital Cryosurgical Center of Southern California, for helping me to gather the information included here on cryosurgery, as well as the Cryosurgery Consent Form.

4. Hypothermia is excessive, possibly dangerous, cooling of the body.

5. Sloughing is a separation or shedding of live tissue from dead tissue.

6. Orandi A. Transurethral resection versus transurethral incision of the prostate. *Urol Clin North Am*. Aug 1990;17(3):601–612.

7. Kletscher BA, Oesterling JE. Transurethral incision of the prostate: A viable alternative to transurethral resection. *Semin Urol*. Nov 1992;10(4): 265–272.

8. Lepor H, Sypherd D, Machi G, Derus J. Randomized double-blind study comparing the effectiveness of balloon dilatation of the prostate and cystoscopy for the treatment of symptomatic benign prostatic hyperplasia. *J Urol*. Mar 1992;147(3):639–642; discussion 642–644.

9. Laduc R, Bloem FA, Debruyne FM. Transurethral microwave thermotherapy in symptomatic benign prostatic hyperplasia. *Eur Urol.* 1993; 23(2):275–281.

6 Other Standard Treatments for Prostate Problems

1. *Physicians' Desk Reference,* 1994 edition, Oradell, NJ: Medical Economics Company: p 2639.
2. See Chapter 8 for a discussion of Gleason scores.
3. Haim Bicher, M.D., the head of the Valley Cancer Institute in Los Angeles, contributed much of the information on hyperthermia.
4. Kei TK, et al., of the College of Physicians, Columbia University, April 2, 1986, as quoted in *Cancer Victims Journal.* Summer-Fall 1988;22(2 & 3): 5.
5. Fleming C, et al. A decision analysis of alternative treatment strategies for clinically localized prostate cancer. *JAMA.* May 26, 1993;20:2650–2658. Whitmore, WF. Management of clinically localized prostate cancer. (editorial) *JAMA.* May 26, 1993;20:2676–2670.

7 Alternative Approaches to Treating the Prostate

1. Buck AC, et al. Treatment of outflow tract obstruction due to benign prostatic hyperplasia with the pollen extract, Cernilton. *Br J Urol.* 1990; 66:398–404.
2. Rugendorff EW, et al. Results of treatment with pollen extract (Cernilton® N) in chronic prostatitis and prostatodynia. *Br J Urol.* 1993;71:433–438.
3. For an overview of the Oriental medicine approach to prostate problems, I spoke to Randy W. Martin, O.M.D., Ph.D., LAc. Dr. Martin is a Doctor of Oriental Medicine and a Licensed Acupuncturist practicing in Encino, California.

8 If the Diagnosis Is Cancer

1. From the American Cancer Society Cancer Response System, #462557.
2. Adapted from Catalona, WJ. Management of cancer of the prostate. *N Eng J Med.* 1994;331:996–1004.
3. Levy JA. Nutrition and the immune system, in Sites DP, et al. *Basic and Clinical Immunology.* 4th ed. Los Altos, CA: Lange Medical Publications, 1982, pp 297–305.
4. See Chandra RK. Nutrition and immunity—Basic considerations. Part 1. *Contemporary Nutrition* 11(11), 1986: Levy, JA. Nutrition and the immune system, in Sites DP, et al. *Basic and Clinical Immunology.* 4th ed. Los Altos, CA: Lange Medical Publications, 1982, pp. 297–305.

5. See Chandra RK. Nutrition and immunity—Basic considerations. Part 1. *Contemporary Nutrition* 11(11), 1986: Alexander M, et al. Oral beta-carotene can increase the number of OKTA4+ cells in human blood. *Immunology Letters.* 1985;9:221–224.

6. Chandra RK, 1986, ibid.

7. Chandra RK, 1986, op cit.

8. Prinz W, et al. The effect of ascorbic acid supplementation on some parameters of the human immunological defense system. *International Journal of Vitamin Nutrition Research.* 1977;47(3):248–257.

9. See Beisel WR, et al. Single nutrient effects on immunologic functions. *JAMA.* 1981;245(1):53–58. Chandra RK, 1986: Levy JA, 1982.

10. Chandra RK, 1986, op cit.: Chandra RK, Trace element regulation of immunity and infection. *J Am Coll. Nut.* 1985;4(1):5–16.

11. See Chandra RK, 1986; Chandra RK, 1985: Levy JA, 1982.

12. Levy JA, 1982.

13. See Levy JA, 1982, op cit.: Chandra RK, Trace element regulation of immunity and infection. *J Am Coll. Nut.* 1985;4(1):5–16.

14. Chandra RK, 1986, op cit.: Chandra RK, 1985, op cit.

15. Mettlin C, et al. Vasectomy and prostate cancer risk. *Am J Epidemiology.* 1990;132(6):1056–1061.

16. Rosenberg L, et al. Vasectomy and the risk of prostate cancer. *Am J Epidemiology.* 1990;132(6):1051–1055.

9 Dealing with the Serious Side Effects of Prostate Problems

1. To learn about HIP or to obtain more information about the treatment of incontinence, contact HIP at P.O. Box 544, Union, SC, 29379. Or call 1-800-BLADDER.

2. Adapted from the Brief Pain Inventory (Short Form), *Management of Cancer Pain: Adults, Quick Reference Guide for Clinicians.* Number 9, U.S. Department of Health and Human Services, Public Health Service. Agency for Health Care Policy and Research. AHCPR Publication No. 94-0593, March 1994, pp 24–25.

10 Honest Talk from Men Who Have Been through It

1. Dole R. Of cancer and candor. *People Magazine.*

2. Maugh TH. The disease men try to ignore. *Los Angeles Times,* Jan 2, 1995; p A1.

3. Reprinted with permission from the authors from US TOO, June/July 1993.

11   The Healthy Prostate Program, Part I: Prevention

1. Holden JM, et al. Zinc and copper self-selected diets. *J Am Dietetic Assoc.* 1979;75:25.

2. Elsborg L, et al. The intake of vitamins and minerals by the elderly at home. *Inst. J. Vit Nutrit Res.* 1983;53:321–329.

3. Personal communication, Seymour Ehrenpreis, November 11, 1994.

4. For more on DLPA, see Fox A & Fox B. *DLPA to End Chronic Pain and Depression.* New York: Simon & Schuster, 1985.

12   The Healthy Prostate Program, Part II: Treatment

1. See Chapter 3 for a discussion of the culture and sensitivity.

2. Catalona WJ. Management of cancer of the prostate. *N Eng J Med.* 1995;331:998.

3. Diethylstibestrol, 1 to 3 mg by mouth daily.

4. Leuprolide acetate, depot dose, 7.5 mg intramuscularly, once a month; or Goserelin acetate implant, 3.5 mg subcutaneously, once a month.

5. 250 mg, 3 times a day.

13   The Latest Word on Treating the Prostate

1. Osterling JE. Benign prostatic hyperplasia: Medical and minimally invasive treatment options. *New Eng J Med.* 1995;332(2):99–109.

2. "Percutaneous cryosurgery for prostate surgery." Joan Stephenson. *Internal Medicine News,* February 15, 1995, p 5.

3. Osterling, op cit., p100.

4. "Prostate-specific antigen density testing debated." *Medical Tribune,* February 2, 1995, p 4.

5. "Needle biopsy DNA analysis helps predict prostate cancer recurrence." *Internal Medicine News,* January 15, 1995, p 1.

Glossary

acute bacterial prostatitis A sudden and/or severe inflammation of the prostate, associated with bacteria. It responds well to antibiotics.

adenoma A benign (noncancerous) tumor of glandular epithelium (like the lining of the stomach).

AIDS Acquired immunodeficiency syndrome. Apparently caused by the human immunodeficiency virus (HIV), AIDS attacks the immune system, weakening the body's defenses. AIDS itself does not seem to kill us, but it ruins the immune system, leaving us helpless prey to other diseases.

benign prostatic hypertrophy (BPH) An unwanted and unnecessary growth of the prostate that can cause urinary and other problems. BPH is *not* cancerous.

benign tumor A tumor that grows slowly and does not metastasize (spread). It may obstruct, interfere with, or pressure other body tissue. A benign tumor is *not* a cancer.

biopsy Removal of a small piece of tissue from the body for examination. The piece of tissue itself is referred to as the biopsy specimen.

cancericidal Something that kills cancer cells and is used in chemotherapy and other approaches to battling cancer. Your body produces many cancer-killers, such as the natural killer cells of the immune system.

carcinoma Cancer, although the term carcinoma is usually applied to groups of cancers that develop on coverings and linings in the body (such as the lining of the stomach).

chlamydia A bacterial infection that can infect the prostate. Chlamydia can cause sterility in men and women, ectopic pregnancies in women, and other problems in both sexes. It can be treated with antibiotics.

chronic bacterial prostatitis   A less-severe inflammation of the prostate, associated with bacteria. The symptoms may come and go. Does not respond well to medicines.

cysto-, cyst-, cysti-   Prefixes referring to the bladder.

cystography   A test involving the infusion of dye into the bladder so that X rays may be taken.

cystoscope   A long, thin instrument with lenses that is used to examine and treat the bladder and ureter.

cystoscopy   Inserting a cystoscope into the urethra in order to visually examine the lower urinary tract.

epididymitis   An acute or chronic inflammation of the epididymis.

genital warts   A condition caused by the human papilloma virus (HPV). They have been associated with cervical and possibly penile cancer. They are considered dangerous. Genital warts are highly contagious and must be treated immediately.

gonorrhea   A contagious inflammation of the genital mucous membrane caused by a bacteria. Gonorrhea can be cured with antibiotics. If not treated, gonorrhea can infect other parts of the body, and can cause urethral stricture, prostatitis, sterility, arthritis, and skin sores.

herpes   An inflammatory viral disease of the skin and mucous membrane. Herpes I usually produces cold sores around the mouth, while herpes II produces outbreaks in the genital area. The diseases are chronic, but not deadly. Herpes may remain dormant within the body for years, then suddenly flare up. A cure has not yet been developed.

leukemia   A cancer of the blood.

malignant tumor   A fast-growing tumor that invades other parts of the body, either directly or by metastasis. A malignant tumor *is* a cancer.

metastasize   To spread to other parts of the body.

neoplasm   A new growth, an abnormal mass that serves no useful purpose and grows at the expense of other cells.

nonbacterial prostatitis   A disease that causes symptoms similar to those of bacterial prostatitis, but for which no cause can be found. Drug therapy is not effective.

orchitis   An inflammation of one or both testes.

prostate cancer   Uncontrolled and potentially deadly growth of the prostate tissue. Prostate cancer can cause urinary and, possibly, sexual difficulties. It becomes deadly only when it spreads beyond the prostate gland.

prostatitis   An inflammation of the prostate that causes a variety of symptoms, including urgency, increased frequency of urination, increased frequency of nighttime urination, difficulty in urinating, pain upon urinating and/or ejaculating, plus other pains and problems. There are three types of prostatitis: acute bacterial prostatitis, chronic bacterial prostatitis, and nonbacterial prostatitis.

prostatodynia   Pain that seems to originate in the prostate but has other causes (such as origin in the muscle).

prostatostasis   Problem caused by an inability of prostatic fluid to drain properly. Chronic nonbacterial prostatitis is sometimes called prostatostasis.

retrograde   Backward, or to go back over. In retrograde ejaculation, the sperm goes up toward the bladder rather than down the urethra.

sarcoma   Cancers of the bone, muscle, and connective tissue. Less common than carcinomas.

syphilis   A contagious venereal disease caused by the spirochete, *Treponema pallidum*. Syphilis can be treated with antibiotics. If not treated, it can damage the brain, heart, spinal cord, and other parts of the body, leading to blindness, insanity, and death.

tumor   An abnormal, new growth that serves no useful purpose, does not work with other cells for the good of the body, and grows at the expense of other cells.

urethritis   An inflammation of the ureter, the tube that carries urine from the bladder out of the body. Not a prostate problem at all, but may produce similar symptoms.

urethro-   A prefix referring to the urethra.

urethrography   A test involving the infusion of dye into the urethra so that X rays may be taken.

urethroscope   A thin instrument with lenses used to visually examine the urethra.

urethroscopy   Inserting a special instrument into the urethra in order to examine it visually.

For Further Reading

Adler J: The killer we don't discuss. *Newsweek* 1993 Dec 27,p40(2).

Assessing need for repeated biopsies. *USA Today* (magazine) 1993 Feb, p13(1).

Balloon treatment avoids surgery. *USA Today* (magazine) 1990 Oct,p12(1).

Benderly B: Grand illusion: there's a killer stalking American men. But are they man enough to defeat it? *Amer Health* 1990 Dec,p68(5).

Berries for the prostate? *Consumer Reports* 1994 Mar,p207(1).

Bowers J: Adieu, old pal. *Amer Health* 1992 Oct,p62(2).

Carey B: The prostate predicament. *Health* 1994 May–Jun,p101(4).

Carlson R: The other prostate problem (benign prostate hyperplasia). *Amer Health* 1992 Oct,p59(4).

Cicero K: No-knife cancer cure (radiation treatment). *Health* 1991 Feb, p20(1).

Cowley G: Rethinking prostate surgery: The search is on for alternative to the knife. *Newsweek* 1991 Aug 5,p48(1).

———— : To test or not to test. *Newsweek* 1993 Dec 27,p42(2).

Dittman R Jr: Help for the disease men fear most. *Reader's Digest* 1992 Dec,p209(6).

Does sex help the prostate? *Consumer Reports* 1993 Nov,p743(1).

Dunn D: Prostate cancer: How to thwart a killer. *Business Week* 1992 Mar 16,p132(2).

Fackelmann K: Large prostate? New drug provides relief. *Science News* 1991 Jun 8,p357(1).

Fox A and Fox B. *Beyond Positive Thinking*. Carson, CA: Hay House, 1991.

————. *DLPA to End Chronic Pain and Depression*. New York: Pocket Books, 1985.

————. *Immune for Life*. Rocklin, CA: Prima Publishing, 1989.

————. *Making Miracles*. Emmaus, PA: Rodale Press, 1989.

Gorman C: The private pain of prostate cancer. *Time* 1992 Oct 5,p77(2).

Gutfeld G, et al: Choosing your best prostate prescription. *Prevention* 1994 Jun,p80(14).

————— , et al: Rays of remedy: sun-induced vitamin D linked to less prostate cancer. *Prevention* 1993 Jun,p14(2).

Kaltenbach D with Richards T. *Prostate Cancer. A Survivor's Guide.* New Port Richey, FL: Seneca House Press, 1995.

Kirtz F, et al: Pills instead of prostate surgery. *U.S. News & World Report* 1991 Jun 17,p66.

Kreiter T: A new believer in early detection. *Saturday Evening Post* 1993 May–Jun,p14(2).

Laliberte R: The prostate debate. *Men's Health* 1993 Dec,p65(5).

Lawren B: A wife's guide to prostate problems. *Good Housekeeping* 1992 Mar,p98(1).

Lax E: Is your husband dying of embarrassment? The truth about prostate cancer. *Family Circle* 1993 July20,p57(4).

Lend the gland a hand: Exercise lowers risk for prostate cancer. *Prevention* 1992 Aug,p10(2).

Lipsyte R: Hot gland. *Amer Health* 1994 Mar,p28(2).

Mann C: The prostate-cancer dilemma. *The Atlantic* 1993 Nov,p102(12).

Martin W. *My Prostate and Me. Dealing with Prostate Cancer.* New York: Cadell & Davies, 1994.

Maugh TH: The disease men try to ignore. *Los Angeles Times*, Jan 2, 1995, pA1.

Meyer S and Nash S. *Prostate Cancer. Making Survival Decisions.* Chicago: The University of Chicago Press, 1994.

Mobilizing for early prostate cancer detection. *Saturday Evening Post* 1992 Sep–Oct,p56(2).

Nash JM: Stopping cancer. New discoveries about wayward genes and misbehaving proteins show how cells become malignant—and perhaps how to bring them under control. *Time* 1994 Apr 25,p54(7).

New prostate test. *Consumer Reports* 1991 Nov,p717(1).

Newman R: Chilling prostate cancer. *U.S. News & World Report* 1992 Oct 12,p84(2).

Phillips R. *Coping with Prostate Cancer: A practicing psychologist offers meaningful, sound, and compassionate advice to those who must deal with prostate cancer.* Garden Park City, New York: Avery Publishing Group, 1994.

Podolsky D: Big claims, no proof. *U.S. News & World Report* 1991 September 23:77.

————— , et al: Heal thyself. *U.S. News & World Report* 1993 Nov 22,p64(7).

————— : Should you get tested? *U.S. News & World Report* 1992 May 4, p74(2).

Polevo M: High-tech cancer tests. *Amer Health* 1992 Sep,p9(3).

Prostate cancer: Conspiracy of silence. *U.S. News & World Report* 1992 May 11,p68(2).

Prostate cancer may have roots in genetic defect. *Los Angeles Times*, Nov 22, 1994,pA30.

Prostate problems after dark (enlarged prostate can lead to an overdistended bladder). *Consumer Reports* 1993 Sept,p580(1).

The prostate puzzle. *Consumer Reports* 1993 Jul,p459(1).

Prostate screening can be risky. *USA Today* (magazine) 1991 Oct,p7(1).

PSA and age. *Reader's Digest* 1994 Apr,p129(1).

Radioactive iodine curbs cancer. *USA Today* (magazine) 1992 Oct,p12(2).

Rous S. *The Prostate Book. Sound Advice on Symptoms and Treatment.* New York: W.W. Norton & Co., 1994.

Slon S: Man trouble. *Men's Health* 1993 Mar–Apr,p32(3).

The need for cancer screening. *USA Today* (magazine) 1990 Feb,p12(1).

Thornton J: Pharm aid: 10 new medicines you should know about. *Men's Health* 1990 Oct,p73(5).

Unmasking a stealthy cancer: A simple blood test can boost the detection of prostate tumors. *Time* 1991 May 6,p45(1).

Wake Up! You're Alive. An MD's Prescription for Healthier Living Through Positive Thinking. Deerfield Beach, FL: Health Communications, 1988.

Walter R. *Options. The Alternative Cancer Therapy Book.* New York: Avery Publishing Group, 1993.

What if it's cancer. *Consumer Reports* 1993 Jul,p463(3).

When the prostate swells. *Consumer Reports* 1993 Jul,p469(3).

Wickens B: Middle-age suffering. *Maclean's* 1992 Mar 16,p45(1).

Index